The *Smart Woman's*
Guide to Diabetes

Authentic Advice on Everything From
Eating to Dating and Motherhood

The *Smart Woman's* Guide to Diabetes

Authentic Advice on Everything From Eating to Dating and Motherhood

Amy Stockwell Mercer

demosHEALTH

New York

Visit our website at www.demoshealth.com

ISBN: 978-1-936303-13-7

E-book ISBN: 9781617050701

Acquisitions Editor: Noreen Henson

Compositor: Absolute Service, Inc.

Printer: Bang Printing

Library of Congress Cataloging-in-Publication Data

CIP data is available from the Library of Congress.

Special discounts on bulk quantities of Demos Health books are available to corporations, professional associations, pharmaceutical companies, healthcare organizations, and other qualifying groups. For details, please contact:

Special Sales Department
Demos Medical Publishing
11 West 42nd Street, 15th Floor
New York, NY 10036
Phone: 800–532–8663 or 212–683–0072
Fax: 212–941–7842
E-mail: rsantana@demosmedpub.com

Made in the United States of America

11 12 13 14 / 5 4 3 2

*This book is dedicated to the four men
in my life: my husband Dale,
and my three amazing sons,
Will, Miles, and Reid.*

Contents

Foreword

As a woman who has lived with diabetes for more than two decades, I have performed my fair share of literary searches for books that would guide me through various life stages: puberty, college life, dating, marriage, pregnancy, and parenting. There were the typical difficulties of the college years that included sitting in my dorm room tearfully trying to figure out how and where to wear my new insulin pump under my form-fitting party dress. There was also the question that goes though the mind of every single woman with diabetes, "When should I tell a love interest about my diabetes? On the first date? After he (or she) meets my family? What is proper protocol and what do other women with diabetes do?" Eventually there was the very lonely experience of pregnancy with diabetes. I had no idea what was normal or what to expect. "Did that blood sugar of 242 mg/dL hurt my baby? What will my blood sugar do during delivery? Should I wear my insulin pump when I'm in labor or not?"

Unfortunately, my literary searches on these topics were usually disappointing. In fact, *The Diabetic Woman* by Lois Jovanovic served as my only resource on such gender-specific diabetes topics for as long as I can recall. Although Jovanovic's book will always serve as a classic in many women's home libraries (including my own), I was overjoyed to learn about, and honored to be a part of, *The Smart Woman's Guide to Diabetes*. To say this book is long overdue is an understatement. For far too long, the unique needs and experiences of women with diabetes have been overlooked. I am excited to see inspiring women like Amy Mercer step up to shine a spotlight on the these issues that not only help women with diabetes, but also raise the public's awareness. As women with diabetes, we have gained incredible strength through the trials and tribulations that are unique to us. We have learned important lessons that are invaluable to other women with diabetes. That kind of real life, practical advice from peers is priceless. I thank Amy for compiling this information to help me and millions of other women through various life stages. No matter what stage of life you are in, if you are a woman with diabetes, this book will help you navigate each stage with sound, practical advice from your peers with diabetes. If you are like me and you spent many years dreaming of having a friend with diabetes to talk to or relate to, this book will be your "ultimate girl-friend with diabetes." A friend to provide great guidance and advice throughout every stage of life.

It seems that Amy and I were destined to be a part of each other's lives. God brings people into our lives for various reasons. Sometimes we know why that person is there and other times we do not. The connection between me and Amy was immediate because the purpose of our lives is so similar. We are true "DiabetesSisters" with kindred spirits. While *my* work with women with diabetes has focused on web and in-person programming at DiabetesSisters, *Amy's* work has focused on print resources. Our goals are very similar; to reduce the isolation felt by so many women with diabetes. This cause is incredibly personal to both of us because we have felt the sting of loneliness in our own diabetes experiences.

Throughout my work in diabetes during the past 15 years and my work specifically with women with diabetes over the past four years, I have met few people as passionate and determined to help women with diabetes as Amy. We met years ago when DiabetesSisters was a fledgling organization and had just applied for federal nonprofit status. We were a true grassroots organization whose only form of advertise-ment was word-of-mouth. Amy contacted me as soon as she learned about DiabetesSisters and expressed her appreciation for the resource as well as her desire to contribute to such an important cause. Her pas-sion for serving women with diabetes was immediately obvious. From the beginning, I identified her as a woman who really understood what DiabetesSisters was all about. Through her desire to help other women with diabetes she served as a type 1 blogger on the DiabetesSisters website in 2008, has participated in the Weekend for Women Confer-ence series, and is leading a new PODS Meetup (support group) in her own town of Charleston, South Carolina.

In our first conversation in 2008, I vividly recall Amy sharing her dream of writing a book that would educate and support women with diabetes throughout their life's journey with this disease. To her credit, I have talked to many people over the past few years who have shared their bigger-than-life dreams with me, but I can count on one hand the number of those people who were passionate and determined enough to follow through on their dream. From one woman who has followed her dream to another, I say, "Well done, phenomenal woman!" From one DiabetesSister to another who has followed her dream to support and educate other women with diabetes, I say, "Outstanding work, inspiring sister!"

Brandy Barnes
Founder/CEO
DiabetesSisters

Acknowledgments

I'd like to thank my mom Teddy Stockwell and step-dad Charley Gibbes for the countless hours they spent with my three boys so that I could have time to write. I also want to thank my mom for inspiring my love for reading, and for her unwavering and unconditional support. I would like to thank my dad Rick Stockwell for teaching me the value of story-telling, and the importance of following my passion.

This book was built by a team of amazing women who shared their personal and private stories with me about life with diabetes. Thank you: Amy Tenderich, Andie Dominick, Annie Berger, Ann Rosenquist Fee, Andrea McDowell, Brandy Barnes, Cara Bauer, Cheryl Alkon, Emily Wefelmeyer, Heather Schlesinger, Heather Jacobs, Holly Witteman, Jennifer Ahn, Jessica Apple, Judith Jones Ambrosini, Katie McCutcheon, Katie Savin, Kathleen Fraser, Kelly Love Johnson, Kristin Makszin, Laura Bennett, Lee Ann Thill, Lesley Hoffman Goldenberg, Linda Frick, Lori Dubrow, Maia Caemmerer, Mallory Boyd, Mari Ruddy, Melinda Law, Michelle Sorensen, Rachel Garlinghouse, Rebecca Walker Bryant, Sarah Howard, Sloan Wesloh, Stella Biggs, and Vicki Taniwaki.

More thanks go out to the professional women who took the time to talk to me and share their wisdom about living well with diabetes: Andi Kravitz Weiss, Claire Blum, Janis Roszler, Jessica Bernstein, Lyndsay Riffe, Rosalind Joffee, Margaret Wilkman, Dr. Ann Albright, Dr. Ann Goebel-Fabbri, Dr. Deborah Young-Hyman, Dr. Elizabeth Stephens, Dr. Francine R. Kaufman, Dr. Liana Abascal, Dr. Lois Jovanovic, Dr. Paula M. Trief, and Dr. Sheri Colberg-Ochs.

Thank you to the MFA faculty at Queens University for giving me the confidence to keep going.

And to the doctors, endocrinologists, nutritionists and diabetes educators who have helped me to live well with diabetes.

And to my sister, Erin Grimm, here's to living a long and healthy life with diabetes.

Introduction

Being diagnosed with type 1 diabetes at 14 years old, the cusp of adolescence, changed my life forever. Insulin injections, a "diabetic diet," and the ever-present fear of complications were suddenly added to the typical teenage fixations on boys, clothes, and being popular. Instead of speaking in the 1980s Valley Girl slang, I had to learn a medical dialect—the language of old age. Instead of experimenting with changing hormones and a budding sexuality, I had to learn how to read my body's signals to determine whether I was "high" or "low," whether I needed sugar, or needed to go for a walk to bring my sugar down. All this time, I felt like I was alone, like I was the only one in the world with this dreadful disease.

At 14 years old, I was angry at and scared of my body. I was angry that I had to grow up too soon. I was angry that I was no longer invincible, and that I had a disease that sounded like "die." I wanted to be just like everyone else, and so I shoved my disease deep into the dark and dusty corners of my internal attic. For years, I denied my illness in an attempt to fit in. I couldn't imagine any benefits of living with diabetes. I couldn't conceive that there would be anything that would make this hardship worthwhile. For a long time, I was not strong. I was in denial, and then later, I was bitter.

It's been 25 years since I was diagnosed, and I am now a mother to three healthy boys. I love to spy on my children when they don't know I am there and then listen to their stories. I love the way their imagination works—the way their stuffed animals become real, the songs they sing, and the explorers they become when they play in the marsh near our home. Mostly, I love the fact that their imagination is free from the hard knowledge of reality.

When I began the journey of writing this book, I wondered about my own imagination. I remembered how I used to pretend my name was Jessica or Elizabeth; a girl who had long blonde hair and rode horses. As I grew older, I wrote stories on paper instead of keeping them in my head, and I was always someone different from myself—someone richer, prettier, more popular, more adventurous, and not sick. Looking back, I wondered how many times throughout the 25 years of my life with diabetes have I imagined myself without it. How many times have I wondered if I would be less serious, less controlled, and less bitter? Without diabetes, would I be a more carefree woman?

Several months ago, I came across a story written by a fellow diabetic writer, Riva Greenberg, about living with diabetes as a woman. Her words stopped me cold. She wrote:

> *When life throws us a curve ball like diabetes, or any other challenge, it is up to us how we choose to see it and what we do about it. Do we see a possible gift in what we've been handed and perhaps use our challenge to develop greater strength and courage, or do we only see that we've been injured?*[1]

I realized that it was time for me to look beyond my injuries. I realized that without diabetes, I wouldn't have this story to tell. This story that has turned into a book; a how-to guide about how a woman lives with diabetes. A book that will include the kind of stories I have wanted to hear for years, stories from women telling the good and the bad of this disease. Stories from women who count their blessings, like Heather Jacobs who said, "Today, I have a much different view of diabetes, which I happily share with my fellow diabetes community. First, diabetes IS NOT a death sentence. In fact, if we embrace the lifestyle we then have the potential to live a longer healthier life." Another story is from a young woman named Kayla, who is filled with anger and frustration and says no one knows what it is truly like to live with this disease.

I didn't realize when I started writing this book 5 years ago that I was embarking on a journey that is both emotional and physical. Listening to Kayla and Heather and nearly a hundred other women has allowed me to see that I am not alone. Listening to the stories of women living with diabetes; women who were different from me in terms of age and personality; women who live in different parts of the country and even across the world; women who were athletes, doctors, educators, mothers, and writers; and women who were single, married, and widowed has taught me that I am not alone. We all share the same disease and we all want to know if there are others out there like us. I hope you will join me on this journey of discovery.

1   Diagnosis

Standing in the bathroom in the middle of the night, I gulped water from a plastic cup that was left at the sink. I'd been dreaming about water. At 14 years old, I was living away from home at a boarding school in New Hampshire. In the dark bathroom, while everyone else was sleeping, I was scared of my thirst.

The next morning, my body was heavy and my eyes were slow to open. All I wanted to do was to sleep. However, it was time for school, and my roommate told me that I am going to be late for class if I didn't get out of bed. I told her to go ahead without me. As the October sun streamed through the flimsy curtains of our sole window, I imagined myself standing at the counter of the mini-mart across the street and buying a Diet Cherry Coke or a strawberry-banana milkshake from the den or just water; I could see a glass of water in my mind and I needed water. My thirst got me out of bed.

It was a warm fall day, I walked along the dirt road from my dorm, past the football field, to the white, wooden health center. Dizzily, I opened the door and held onto the edge of the nurse's desk. I listened to another student who was describing her symptoms: achy head, sore throat, and tiredness. The nurse explained to the student that there was a cold going around and then dispensed a travel pack of Tylenol. I didn't have an achy head or a sore throat, but I was tired, so I asked the nurse if blurred vision is a symptom of the cold.

"Yes," she said, "blurred vision is a symptom of the cold." She gave me Tylenol and a note to excuse me from my class. I wasn't used to being sick, other than for a few bouts of strep throat and an occasional allergic reaction that caused my eyes to swell; I've never even had chicken pox. Being sick was a sign of weakness in our family, a sign of being needy, and neediness was bad.

My mouth was still dry that afternoon, and I returned to the health center. "Something's wrong," I told the nurse. While weighing me, she asked me why I lost 15 lbs since I'd been in school. I just shrugged. I hadn't noticed. Following her down the hallway to a sick room, I crawled into bed with a sigh of relief. She pulled the door behind her and I let go of the tension I'd been holding in my jaw. I could hear the faraway noise of my classmates walking by the health center. The room was dark, the shades were drawn, and the bed next to me was empty. I didn't belong there in the darkness; I belonged out there with my classmates. But it was a relief to give in and let go.

In the quiet hum of the infirmary, I heard the nurse's voice on the phone asking to speak with Teddy Stockwell, my mother.

"We think you should come and pick up your daughter. We think she may be anorexic," she said.

I was stunned but relieved. Mom was on her way.

My mom told me that she knew what was wrong the minute she leaned down to kiss me and smelled my sweet breath. My younger sister had been diagnosed with type 1 diabetes 6 months before, and she recognized the symptoms but didn't want to scare me. She hoped that she was wrong.

"Where are we going?" I asked her as we drove away from my school.

"The hospital," she answered. By the time we arrived, my blood sugar was 400 mg/dl. I had type 1 diabetes.

STATISTICS FOR WOMEN AND DIABETES

- Approximately 12.6 million women have diabetes
- 5% to 10% have type 1 diabetes
- 90% to 95% have type 2 diabetes
- 2% to 10% have gestational diabetes
- From 1990 to 1998, diabetes rates have increased to 70% for women aged 30 to 39 years old.

Source: Centers for Disease Control and Prevention (CDC) National Diabetes Fact Sheet, 2011 and Diabetes and Women's Health Across the Life Stages report.

Signs and Symptoms of Diabetes

The signs and symptoms of diabetes can be similar for both types, but they generally develop slower in those with type 2.

1. Frequent urination
2. Unquenchable thirst
3. Weight loss
4. Hunger
5. Fatigue
6. Headaches
7. Blurred vision
8. Chronic yeast infections
9. Sweet breath
10. Numbness in feet
11. Mood swings
12. Tightness of breathing
13. Bedwetting

Diabetes is a big umbrella term. Think of it as a triangle that widens to encompass the various types of diabetes. There is a great deal of controversy with the labels type 1 and type 2 because they share the same name but are different diseases.

Type 1 diabetes is usually diagnosed in children and young adults. In type 1, the body no longer produces insulin. Insulin is a hormone that is needed to convert sugar, starches, and other food into energy that is needed by the body. People with type 1 diabetes need to have multiple daily injections or wear an insulin pump to manage their blood sugar levels.

Type 2 diabetes is the most common form of diabetes. Millions of Americans have been diagnosed with type 2 diabetes, and many more are unaware that they are at risk. Some groups have a higher risk for developing type 2 diabetes, including African Americans, Latinos, Native Americans, Asian Americans, Native Hawaiians and other Pacific Islanders, as well as the aged population. In type 2 diabetes, either your body does not produce enough insulin, or your cells ignore the insulin. Women with type 2 diabetes can manage blood sugar with exercise and diet. However, some people with type 2 diabetes eventually need to inject insulin or wear an insulin pump.

Latent autoimmune diabetes in adults (LADA), sometimes known as type 1.5 diabetes, is diagnosed in adults who are older than 30 years old. LADA is often misdiagnosed as type 2 diabetes because of the age at which individuals develop this condition; however, people with LADA do not have insulin resistance like those with type 2 diabetes. LADA is characterized by age, a lack of family history of type 2 diabetes, a gradual increase in insulin requirements, positive antibodies, and a decreasing ability to make insulin as indicated by a low C-peptide. However, most people with LADA can still produce their own insulin when first diagnosed, like those with type 2 diabetes. In the early stages of the disease, women do not require insulin injections. Instead, they can control their blood glucose levels with meal planning, physical activity, and oral diabetes medications. However, several years after diagnosis, women with LADA must take insulin to control blood glucose levels. During pregnancy, usually at around 28 weeks or later, many women are diagnosed with *gestational diabetes*. A diagnosis of gestational diabetes doesn't mean that a woman had diabetes before she conceived, or that she will have diabetes after giving birth. However, it's important to follow a doctor's advice regarding blood sugar levels and eat a healthy diet during the pregnancy for optimal health.

GETTING YOUR DIAGNOSIS AS A KID

DIAGNOSIS OF DIABETES IN CHILDHOOD

According to recent trends, the diagnosis of diabetes in children and young adults is on the rise:

- Approximately 15,600 youths are diagnosed with type 1 diabetes in the United States each year, about 1 in every 400 to 600 children
- Approximately 3,600 youths are diagnosed with type 2 diabetes each year

Source: Centers for Disease Control and Prevention (CDC) National Diabetes Fact Sheet, 2011 and Diabetes and Women's Health Across the Life Stages report.

Being diagnosed with diabetes can occur at any age, and reactions to the diagnosis are as varied as the women who contract the disease. Some girls remember acccepting and adjusting to the diagnosis quickly, whereas others were worried about being different from the other kids. Heather Schlesinger's parents kept her diagnosis when she was 5 years old from becoming a big deal.

> *I think that one advantage of being diagnosed with diabetes at a young age is that I don't really remember life before my diagnosis. Looking back, I realize that I was fortunate enough to have parents and family who made sure that my life was no different than any other kid or teenager. I don't remember a time in my elementary, middle, or high school education where I was not part of at least one sports team, more specifically soccer and softball. Fruit-punch-flavored Gatorade became a staple to my athletic gear, and my mother was determined to make sure every coach knew that having diabetes was no threat to my athletic performance— and it wasn't. I went to 4 years of sleep-away camp, where I was often the only child with diabetes. But that was never a big deal to me and, therefore, my diabetes was never a "big deal" with the friends I had. In fact, my friends at camp would often ask me to "pretend my sugar was low," so that I could go to the infirmary at night and return to the bunk with lots of snacks for everyone to eat. When I attended sleepover parties in elementary school, my mother would quietly come over in the morning before we ate breakfast to do my shot, and would often leave before anyone noticed she was there. My parents' goal was to normalize my life as much as possible—and they have succeeded.*

Holly Witteman was 7 years old when she was diagnosed with type 1 diabetes and remembers being "pretty unfazed by the whole thing." However, being diagnosed at a young age isn't easy for everyone. Judith Jones Ambrosini believed that she was invincible until her diagnosis.

> *I was a healthy kid except for the occasional twisting an ankle while jumping "Double Dutch" or getting scrapes from tipping over on my bicycle. When I was 7 or 8, I had my tonsils removed. That was my health record.*
>
> *Things changed in October 1962, after a couple of very cold days of surfing in the chilly Atlantic Ocean. I caught a very*

bad cold that wouldn't go away. When I went to the doctor, he diagnosed the flu and the possibility of mononucleosis. All I wanted to do was go home and go to sleep. I was irritable and exhausted. During the night, my older sister came up to my room to see if I needed anything. She couldn't wake me up no matter how hard she tried. She called 911. They rushed me to the ER. All I remember was waking up in a bed that was not mine. It was a hospital bed and a man was standing at the foot of the bed reading a chart. He smiled at me, "How do you feel Miss Jones? You had a rough time." I was very confused. I didn't know what he was talking about and I didn't ask any questions. He assured me I was going to be okay and left. As my mind cleared, I tried to figure out what was wrong and why I was in the hospital. I thought it must have been pneumonia from surfing in bitterly cold temperatures and freezing water. That must be it, pneumonia, I told myself.

Shortly after my self-diagnosis, an aide came into my room with a tray of food. He was very sweet and assured me I'd get used to the "diabetic diet." Diabetic diet? What the hell was he talking about? I thought I had pneumonia. How could I have diabetes? My kid sister Janie had diabetes, not me.

Over the next few days, I learned that my blood glucose had been 1,200 when they brought me in, in a severe diabetic ketoacidosis.

A priest came in to administer last rites. My mother rushed down from Schenectady to New York City. I pulled through though and learned the "orange" method of how to give myself shots.* I drank disgusting NoCal root beer soda, and all my friends from school kept me busy with visits and flowers and jokes. When it was time to be discharged, the doc came in to see if I had any questions. Of course I did. I had one burning question, "Will I still be able to eat hot fudge sundaes?" "Oh no," he replied. When he left the room, I cried for hours. Why bother living? What kind of life could I possibly have without hot fudge sundaes?

---

*The orange method is commonly used to teach people with type 1 diabetes how to inject themselves with a syringe. They are taught to practice on an orange instead of their leg, for example.

DIAGNOSIS DANGERS

Diabetic ketoacidosis (DKA) is a serious condition that can lead to a coma. When cells don't get the glucose they need for energy, the body burns fat that produces ketones or acids that can poison the body.

In her story, Judith expresses the fear and sadness experienced by many young people who are diagnosed with diabetes. Being diagnosed with a chronic illness at any age is a shock—suddenly you are different than you were moments ago—and you'll be different forever. A diagnosis in childhood can put much of the responsibility on the parents. You will hear many of these women share stories of mothers who worked hard to ease their daughter's burden. Lesley Hoffman Goldenberg's mom stood firmly by her side at the hospital when she was diagnosed at 12 years old.

My mom didn't leave my side while I was in the hospital. My brother and sister, who are twins, are 4 years younger than me, so my dad stayed with them. I have this image of my mom from the hospital—she slept next to me on this tiny couch for the entire time I was hospitalized. She had a HUGE stack of books next to the couch where she slept—books on parenting a diabetic child, cooking for a child with diabetes, emotionally supporting a diabetic child, and so on. I remember getting up a lot during the night to use the bathroom and to check my blood sugar—and every single time she was awake either reading or staring at me.

One of the most important things parents can do for their young daughters when they are diagnosed is to let them know that diabetes won't define them. Lesley's story makes this clear:

I think the most important thing they said to us while in the hospital, and a motto my parents implemented in our family, was that we were now a family that had a daughter with diabetes. We were not going to become a diabetic family. We would still travel, go to summer camp, and do

*the same things we always did—life wasn't going to be put
on hold just because of this.*

Women who are diagnosed during adolescence have additional challenges because of hormonal changes. Our bodies are changing physically and emotionally, and most of us, as teenagers, only want to be like
everyone else. Many of the following stories reveal an awareness of
being different as adolescents with diabetes, as well as an understanding of the added responsibility of diabetes management. Many women
struggled to cope with the diagnosis, denying the reality and responsibility of this new identity and being angry because they are no longer
"invincible."

Kayla was 11 years old when she was diagnosed during her school
spring break in Kentucky. She was wetting the bed and very thirsty. Her
mom took her to the Medical University of South Carolina (MUSC), where
doctors said her blood glucose was 600 mg/dl. She stayed at the hospital
for 4 days and couldn't leave until she learned how to do a shot. Kayla
had never heard of diabetes and was very scared. Her first question was,
"Am I going to die?" Her next question was, "Will I have to do a shot?"
She felt like she had to grow up very fast.

> *I got tired of [having diabetes] and I wanted more than
> anything for it to just go away. Now, I'm at the point
> where [I] have completely shut it out of my life. I hardly
> ever check my blood sugars, take insulin, or change my
> sites. I'm past the point of "ignoring" it and I think it's
> more that I have completely forgotten about it. When I sit
> down to eat, the need to check my blood sugar or take
> insulin doesn't even cross my mind. Before, I used to brush
> it off and say, "Oh well!" But now, I don't even remember.
> I've gotten rid of it in a way. No one knows what it's like to
> have diabetes.*

Kayla was sent to a psychiatrist at MUSC because of "adherence"
issues. The doctor suggested Kayla to write a journal entry about her
anger. In it, Kayla wrote:

> *Diabetes upsets me for many different reasons. I wish I
> could be like everyone else and not worry about checking
> my blood sugar, taking insulin, remembering to pack/*

bring extra supplies everywhere, count my carbs at every meal, or change my pump sites. I am a teenager and as if I don't already have enough stress and responsibilities . . . all this extra stuff makes me feel very overwhelmed.

Kayla's denial and frustration are not unusual. There are many young women who struggle every day with accepting this ongoing and demanding disease. However, there are also stories of success, of finding an unexpected strength and resilience within. Lesley Hoffman Goldenberg benefited from a multidisciplinary approach.

Almost immediately, we met with a team comprised of an endocrinologist, a social worker, and a nutritionist. Looking back, it really was the right way to do things. They taught us what diabetes was, how it's treated, how I would have to treat it—but they also addressed the emotional issues and the burden of having this disease.

Annie Berger was diagnosed at 14 years old, and was determined not to let diabetes change her lifestyle.

There was a soccer tournament that I wanted to go to about a week after my diagnosis. I had to prove to my parents that I could take care of myself since I would have to travel alone, and that made me really focus on learning how to take care of myself as quickly as possible (luckily, my coach was a doctor or I don't think they would have let me go). After that, it was back to school and back to my routine of going to practice or games after school and on weekends. I also didn't want to change my life too much around my friends, so I learned how to make diabetes fit into my life. I had a life before my diagnosis, and I worked hard to keep it pretty much the same after.

Hard work is key to successful management and, sometimes, the work can feel overwhelming. Annie continues:

To me, the word diabetes signals a burden. It's a burden to have to think about diabetes all day, every day. It's a burden to have to explain to people, yes I can eat that. It's a burden to deal with having to remember to bring so many supplies with you everywhere you go. And it's a burden to think how it will play a bigger role in my life as I get older and have to begin to deal with the possibility of complications.

When Annie was diagnosed, she didn't know anyone else with diabetes. At 14 years old, she was "too old" for camp, and looking back now, she realized that some kind of support group or camp would have helped her feel less alone. It's important for a child with diabetes to be given the freedom to participate in non-diabetes-related activities (sleepovers and soccer practice) as well as diabetes-focused activities (summer camps, social media websites, blogs, and support groups) to maintain a sense of balance.

My biggest concern after my diagnosis was to get back to school and pick up where I'd left off. Already an outsider because of my small-town upbringing and the fact that I was on financial aid at a school that is largely populated by wealthy kids from Massachusetts and New York, I desperately clung to the loose hold I had on peer acceptance. As the only student at school with diabetes, I quickly shoved my disease into the closet and acted like it was no big deal. However, I remember feeling lonely.

Teenagers with diabetes need to know that they are not alone. Connecting with other teenagers with diabetes can help them feel less isolated or singled out by the disease. Kayla goes to Camp Adam Fisher, a camp for children with diabetes in South Carolina, every summer, and really enjoys the camaraderie. This disease is chronic; it doesn't stop with a diagnosis. The diagnosis is only the beginning.

GETTING YOUR DIAGNOSIS AS AN ADULT

A diagnosis of type 1 or type 2 diabetes or LADA in adult women may be prolonged for various reasons from the business of life, work, school, and/or family, to putting off going to a doctor.

Amy Tenderich, the founder of the award-winning Diabetes Mine website, says her husband had to practically force her to go to the doctor. When Amy got sick, she had a 5-month-old baby, two older children, and was run-down and exhausted. Her life was busy, there was too much to do, her baby was sick, her husband was working long hours, and she didn't have time to go to the doctor. But when she realized that she was waking up weighing less than the day before, she got scared. "I thought, oh my God, this is not right. Is this cancer?"

Amy's husband finally convinced her to go to the doctor who tested her urine and gave a tentative diagnosis of diabetes. "My head was spinning. I thought what? That wasn't even on my list of worries. I didn't know anything about diabetes in adults. I was shocked by the diagnosis, speechless, and scared because that's what my dad died from." Amy went home and put the kids to bed. Suddenly, the phone rang and the lab's staff said that she needed to get to the ER right away. Her blood glucose was 840 mg/dl. "It was the worst night of my life," she says.

It took a full year before Amy's life regained some order. She remembers returning home to her family and trying to incorporate her disease into her life. She remembers getting low readings after every meal because the doctors started her on too much insulin, or because she may have been incorrectly diagnosed and was still in the "honeymoon phase," which is common to people with LADA. As a runner, Amy remembers being scared to go for a run because she was afraid of her blood sugar level becoming low, and wondered if she would be able to exercise again.

"The first day [at] home, I sat on the couch and cried. Then I went to the Internet to search for answers." But there were no blogs nor any information about LADA, and Amy wondered, "Where are all the people? It was as if I was the only adult who got this childhood disease." That's how her website, Diabetes Mine, began.

Amy's story illustrates the lack of understanding about the various types of diabetes among medical practitioners and the need for education. Amy's first year as a woman with diabetes could have been so different if she'd been properly educated and supported from the beginning. However, her negative experience has benefited us all because it resulted in Diabetes Mine, which is a great resource for women living with diabetes.

As a medical student, Jennifer Ahn had a different experience with her diagnosis. She recognized the symptoms and, at a professional and intellectual level, she knew what a diagnosis of diabetes meant.

> *But, being a medical student, I blamed the symptoms on studying and not getting enough sleep . . . I was hungry, thirsty, and always going to the restroom. I actually lost a*

lot of weight—deep down I knew something was wrong.
But, previously being overweight, I thought, hey, I'm
always hungry and eating and now losing weight. I was
actually happy to lose the weight without effort.

Weight loss is a common factor in a diagnosis of type 1 diabetes. Many women spoke about the duality of losing weight, which made them happy, combined with the anxiety and worry of feeling sick and not knowing what was wrong—maybe even not wanting to ask what was wrong. Ann Rosenquist Fee was also happy to lose weight.

It was June of 1994. I was 25 years old, and I wanted to get
pregnant. We'd decided it was time. Or, at least, it was time
to find out if it was time. I went to my OB/GYN to get
checked out and to hear something like: All systems go.
Before the exam, during the usual check-in, I mentioned
recent yeast infections, and the doctor began what I know
now is the standard battery of diabetes diagnosis ques-
tions: Was I urinating frequently? I was, at least every
hour. I'd noticed it about a month earlier, camping up
north, still freezing in May, and I'd had to step out of the
tent lots during the night. Had I lost weight? I had. About
20 lbs in the past few months, but that had me down to
115, and I liked how it looked, so I hardly considered it a
problem. I thought maybe I'd just been walking more, if I
thought about it at all.

Frustrations are common in women who are diagnosed as adults with type 1 diabetes, type 2 diabetes, and/or LADA. They have lived a whole life without diabetes, and suddenly, they have to change how they go about doing many things they are used to; suddenly, they have to relearn the basics of how and when to eat, drive, exercise, and listen to their bodies.

Vicki Taniwaki was wrongly diagnosed with type 2 diabetes at 46 years old.

I didn't have any symptoms of type 2 to speak of; people
of Asian extraction typically acquire diabetes at a lower
body weight than any other ethnicity. I knew to be aware
of the possibility only because both [of my] parents and

my only sibling had been diagnosed. I had all of the classic
symptoms—thirst, weight loss, dehydration—but the
possibility of type 1 was never on my radar. Apparently, it
wasn't on the physician's radar either, because it wasn't
until the third blood draw that the endocrinologist decided
the order should include a look at type 1.

Vicki was stunned and relieved with the diagnosis because she finally had an explanation why she had been exercising and eating well for more than 2 years with no effect on her hemoglobin A1c test (a test that measures average blood glucose control over 2 to 3 months). She kept her diagnosis to herself at first because, as she says:

Society lays unbelievable stigma upon chronic illness,
especially when the perception is that the illness could
have been avoided ("if you would just lose weight, that
must mean you ate too much sugar, etc."). When I wasn't
feeling defective, I felt high-maintenance.

Lyndsay Riffe, a nurse who works with people with diabetes, offers some insight into the transition of living as a person with a chronic disease:

Since I work at an endocrinology office, often the patient
has already been diagnosed, and a large percentage have
had type 2 diabetes for several years, and are at the point
where the primary care physician needs assistance from a
specialist. Often, women especially, will remark how they
hadn't been taking care of themselves as well (not compli-
ant with meds, or not following diet) when something
significant is going on in their family—usually an ill
parent or child. If a woman comments about stress in life
with a parent, child, etc. I make sure to comment on taking
care of herself as much as she is taking care of her family.

Lyndsay brings up an important point about women with chronic illness and how we struggle to put ourselves first. Many of us have learned the hard way on how to take care of low and high blood sugar; sometimes, we have to stop taking care of others and take care of our-selves first. This is easier said than done. Whether we are diagnosed as children, teenagers, in our 30s, or beyond, a diagnosis of diabetes is a kind of death for all of us, a death of the person we were, a person without illness, and acceptance comes only when we have gone through the stages of grief.

GRIEVING FOR THE LIFE YOU ONCE HAD

In his book, *The Wounded Storyteller*, Arthur W. Frank writes about the medical community's resistance to "chaos stories"—stories that describe the messiness of illness and ask for an "enhanced tolerance for chaos as part of a life story." He says, "Attempting to push the person out of this wreckage only denies what is being experienced and compounds the chaos."[1] That's why it's very important to acknowledge that we need to grieve for our old lives. Some stages of grief will take longer than others, and with a chronic illness, many women will reexperience these stages at different parts of their life.

Heather Jacobs wasn't allowed to grieve:

> *It was essential that I not only have a "stiff upper lip," but most importantly, I was not allowed to feel sorry for myself. My feelings were irrelevant. It seemed very straightforward for my parents; I had diabetes, therefore, I must do as the doctors told me to do. Period. End of discussion.*

Feelings of grief are common post-diagnosis. The typical stages of grief as defined by Elisabeth Kübler-Ross in her 1969 book, *On Death and Dying,* include denial, anger, bargaining, depression, and acceptance. The stages of grief are not linear and can't be forced. Some people may experience only two, whereas others may experience a roller coaster effect of cycling back and forth before moving through.[2]

Linda Frick, who was diagnosed in 1961 at 8 years old said:

> *I really had no idea what was happening until the nurse came to me a couple of days after my initial hospitalization and told me I couldn't have ice cream anymore. She never said anything positive about my diagnosis. I basically was in denial for the next 18 years.*

Kelly Love Johnson, who was diagnosed at the age of 30, stayed angry:

> *My grief manifested itself as anger, and I was too busy "being in control" to be depressed. I used to get furious at Burger King commercials. I'd rant about what people were feeding their kids. I yelled at the diabetes nutritionist my doctor referred me to. And about a year into my diagnosis, I remember having a mini-breakdown at Harris Teeter. I literally began sobbing, sat down in the middle of the soup aisle, and when a very nice store employee asked if she could help me, I said (through tears) "EVERYTHING HAS CARBS." It was frustrating trying to figure out what I could and could not eat. I keep my net carbs low, I don't eat food with high fructose corn syrup or trans fats. Grocery shopping is like trigonometry sometimes, and I had just reached a breaking point. I experienced a lot of anger and took it out on my family. There are several members of my family with weight issues who did and do not have diabetes. It pissed me off. It also pissed me off that my family seemed incapable of having any event or celebration that didn't involve food.*

Cara Bauer, who was diagnosed at 28 years old, went through the bargaining stage:

> *At first, it was denial. Then anger, bargaining, etc. I found a therapist so I could work on my feelings over this. She equated my diagnosis and my reaction to it as grief of losing my health, like going through the stages of grief as you would a death. In retrospect, I think she was right. I moved through the emotions, but found myself coming back to anger for quite a while. Why, at the age of 28, would I develop this disease? The bargains I remember were kind of silly, actually. I'll take care of myself and live with this disease if I can have a baby. What I remember most was the anger. I was in the anger for a long time. I still return there on occasion.*

DIABETES BLUES

Clinical depression is a reality for 15% to 20% of women living with diabetes. More women experience temporary depression when they first learn their diagnosis. Women with chronic illnesses may struggle with depression throughout their lives, especially as they get older and the risks of complications increase.

Ann Rosenquist Fee wanted to be planning a family, not dealing with a chronic illness.

> *After the hospital, back in our apartment, Scott and I were out of groceries. We went shopping and brought along the lists the diabetes educator had given me. Reading those labels was the most boring, tedious, and daunting thing. I'd never cared before and still didn't care, and didn't want to care, about the nutritional makeup of canned green beans. It was the last thing I wanted to do, to pay attention to that. We bought cheese and Ritz crackers, and back at the apartment, I weighed 2 oz of cheese and cut that in slices on six crackers on a plate. In my messy apartment, on that hot June Sunday afternoon, that stupid plate was the bleakest thing I'd ever seen.*

Rachel Garlinghouse, who was diagnosed when she was 24 years old, went through all the stages of grief:

> *I went through all the stages of grief just like my first certified diabetes educator (CDE) said I would. She told me 3 days after I was diagnosed that I would have to grieve the loss of my body's insulin just like a person grieves the loss of a family member who has died. She was right. But soon, I "put on my big girl panties" and took an active role in my health. Type 1 diabetes is a do-or-die disease. There's no half-doing.*

Kristin Makszin experienced various emotional responses:

> *In the first few days, I was almost excited. I was anxious to read and learn and be the BEST diabetic ever. As time*

*went by, I started to grieve and it came in waves. About
1 week after coming home from the hospital, I had my first
episode where I panicked about what to do with my life
now that I have diabetes. Eventually, I began to accept my
diabetes. Now, it is only a few times a year where I really
feel sorry for myself and overwhelmed by dealing with life
with diabetes.*

*I saw a counselor at my college for the first year. We
actually didn't talk about diabetes too much, but it was
nice to have somewhere to go every week where someone
would ask how I was managing.*

Heather Jacobs experienced a lot of negative feelings and heavy
emotions:

*When asking about how I developed diabetes, I remember
being told something along these lines: I had been on a
cliff, moving toward the edge, when finally the flu pushed
me over the side. It took me years to understand that they
were talking specifically about the destruction of my beta
cells due to autoimmune dysfunction.*

*For me, diabetes was a cursed death sentence. There was
no other option offered other than "you have diabetes, you
will suffer miserable microvascular complications, and
then you will die." I wasn't told that my actions did matter.
I don't know if that would have changed my actions, but it
would have given me at least some hope that I didn't
HAVE to die a slow, agonizing death.*

*Today, I have a much different view of diabetes, which
I happily share with my fellow diabetes community. First,
diabetes IS NOT a death sentence. In fact, if we embrace
the lifestyle, we then have the potential to live a longer,
healthier life compared to those who don't embrace it.
Next, I stress blindness, kidney dysfunction, and nontrau-
matic amputations are NOT complications of diabetes.
Rather, they are potential complications of uncontrolled
diabetes. How we live our lives and embrace our circumstances really does matter.*

Accepting diabetes has a lot to do with being able to talk about diabetes. Diabetes has its own language, one that we slowly become fluent in as the years pass. However, just as new tools to manage the disease are frequently introduced, our language is in a constant state of renewal or transformation. Diabetes slang is used and worn like a badge of honor, but there is an underlying uncertainty about the words we use to describe this disease. Are we diabetics or women with diabetes?

THE LANGUAGE OF ILLNESS

The term *diabetes* was derived from the Greek word for *siphon*, because the water that was drunk by people who were sick with diabetes seemed to run right through their bodies like a siphon. When I was first diagnosed, I hated the word "diabetes." At 14 years old, diabetes sounded like die, and I was suddenly no longer an invincible teenager.

Humor helps, and the following is a list of diabetes slang found on various blogs.

DIABETES SLANG[3]

- **Bouncing.** When your blood sugar drops so low overnight that your body kicks in some glucagons, causing your blood sugar to bounce from low to high
- **Born-again diabetic.** When a person with diabetes fosters a new-found interest in taking care of his or her health after years of negligence and denial
- **Carbonese.** The ability to determine the number of carbs in a given food based on the total carbs and the serving size (coined by a 6-year-old girl with diabetes who is fluent in Carbonese and can eyeball the carbs without her mother's input)
- **Dead strips.** Used blood glucose meter strips found in random spots, such as, under the seat of your car, on the floor at the gym, in a shoe, in the mouth of a small gray kitten named Siah

- **Diabetic PMS.** When the blood sugar rockets up for no apparent reason for the 2 to 3 days prior to the start of a woman's cycle. Men may also experience this in a sympathetic mode.
- **Dotties.** When you squeeze your pricked finger that results in about five holes showing up with blood.
- **Gusher.** When you squeeze your pricked finger, and end up assaulted by your own bloodstream. May also be found when you remove an infusion set.
- **Panicky diabetic syndrome.** The use of more than five test strips in a 55-minute period because you aren't confident that your blood sugar is coming up or down. Often accompanied by a Rage or Serial Bolus.
- **Real-people sick.** The differentiation between blood sugar issues and the common cold. This phrase slips out most often when the person with diabetes admits to not feeling well and must specify that it is not blood-sugar related.
- **Sleep-eating.** The act of rising from a sound sleep, proceeding to the kitchen, and eating anything you find. Persons with diabetes often wake up while in the process of sleep-eating without being able to figure out how they got to the kitchen or why there is ice cream all over their fingers and face.

This confusion about the term *diabetes*, and whether someone is a *diabetic* or is *living with diabetes*, and whether they have type 1, type 2, type 1.5, gestational, or LADA, reflects an ambiguity; what do we have, what does it mean, and how do we define ourselves? The language of illness is very scientific and women are quickly immersed in the challenge of learning a new language after being diagnosed. We are taught that diabetes leads to death, kidney disease, blindness, and amputation. We are taught some phrases such as *combat the illness*, *wage a war against complications*, *battle the disease*, and *control our blood sugar*.

I have never been comfortable with the language of diabetes and have never felt that the terms I used were "right"; for example, the small zippered pouch I use to carry my supplies, I call my "shot bag." However, I don't even give myself shots anymore thanks to the pump, so what should I call it? Am I giving myself shots, or multiple daily injections?

Why, as women with diabetes, do we have to learn to speak like medical professionals to talk about our disease? Is it a disease, an illness, or a chronic condition? If we don't know how to communicate about diabetes, how can we accept it fully into our lives? How can we own it and color it with a pink ribbon, like women with breast cancer, if we don't speak the language?

Heather Jacobs was diagnosed with type 1 diabetes after going into a DKA coma in 1978 at 8 years old. The severity of her health at the time of diagnosis caused her doctors to label her as a "brittle" diabetic. There is debate about whether this is even a correct term, and doctors' and patients' definitions vary widely.

> *My reactions were mixed. On one hand, I felt FINE. I certainly didn't feel like I belonged in the hospital, as that is where people go when they are really sick or injured, and I didn't feel either. On the other hand, I was mentally reeling from what the doctors told me. Simply put: I shouldn't have survived the coma in the first place. What?! I almost died? The doctors followed with an extremely grim prognosis; I had "brittle" juvenile diabetes and had to take shots every day for the rest of my life. I was pissed about calling me "brittle," as I was, in my opinion, one tough kid who prided herself on being able not to cry when hurt. I refused to identify with "brittle," and to this day, I still don't! Lastly, the doctors said I would be dead by age 40, blind, with an amputation, and most likely on dialysis. What was going on? I felt FINE!*

Dr. Elizabeth (Liz) Stephens says, "Language is interesting. There is no other disease like it where every moment of every day is affected by diabetes. Whether you are type 1 or type 2, there is such a diverse population of people with diabetes."

Being able to talk about diabetes also means being able to tell people that you have the disease. Many women have questions about when to tell family, friends, coworkers, significant others, even strangers. When do we tell, who do we tell, and how do we say it?

WORD REPLACEMENT

- Diet   with   Healthy Eating
- Seizure   with   Low
- Restrictions   with   Moderation
- High Risk   with   Specialized
- Complications   with   Challenges
- Brittle   with   Fragile

SHARING THE NEWS AND ASKING FOR HELP

Kelly Love Johnson told her roommate, friends, and coworkers about her type 2 diabetes diagnosis.

> *I think I wanted to wait until I had good news (that the metformin was working, that I wasn't going to be hospitalized). I told close friends next, my roommate (who was wonderful about completely restocking our kitchen and helping me learn how to cook healthy—it was good for him, too), coworkers (but only when one of them saw me test my blood glucose before lunch under my desk at work and told everyone else). It took me about 6 months to be comfortable saying, "No thanks, I don't drink, I'm a diabetic," or "No thanks, I don't eat cake, I'm a diabetic." It's sad to me now to think how hard I was on myself and how much I blamed myself for my disease, and sad that I was alone in the first weeks of my diagnosis because I refused to share it with anyone. But I'm also proud of the fact that I took control of it. I tell people now that my diagnosis saved my life. I believe it did. I think if I hadn't changed my lifestyle, I would have ended up hospitalized with something else (like gallstones, pancreatitis, and other things people I know who are heavy drinkers and poor eaters have gotten). I could have ended up having a heart attack in my 30s.*

I still have some issues. I don't tell "new" friends for a long time. Being in a new city and trying to make friends when you're already the "new" person . . . maybe it is crazy, but I have made friends here—not "best" friends—who still don't know that I don't drink or that I have diabetes. My few close friends here know, and most of them don't really drink either, or at least not heavily. I don't tell men I date that I'm diabetic. I've given it a lot of thought and it isn't because I'm embarrassed; it's because so many people have a preconceived notion of what a "diabetic" is, and I don't want to be treated any differently than anyone else. Believe it or not, there are people who think diabetics cannot have children. Also, I don't want people inviting me to dinner parties and feeling like they have to make "special food"; I don't want coworkers freaking out if I skip lunch. I own this disease, but it's up to me who I share it with.

TIPS ON TELLING OTHERS THAT YOU HAVE DIABETES

Friends and Coworkers:

- Keep it simple. Don't overexplain. Think of sharing this information in the same way as you would share where you grew up, how many kids you have, what you do for fun and, oh yeah, you have diabetes.
- Expect questions, strange reactions, or even no reaction.
- When telling your boss and/or coworkers be prepared to explain that you may need accommodations at work (more on this in Chapter 7).
- Explain what a low blood sugar episode looks like, describe the symptoms, and what they can do to help. People like to be needed and to be asked for help.

Family:
Diabetes is a disease that can affect the whole family from food choices to eating out to helping with low blood sugar. Discussions

with family members will be different than discussions with friends and coworkers.

- Share/suggest a reading material.
- Bring the family to doctor appointments so they can learn from someone other than you and ask questions.
- In the book, *When You're a Parent with Diabetes*, Kathryn Gregorio Palmer (2006) says simply, "Honest statements work best when telling younger children. Read books about diabetes, role play with stuffed animals and with older children, and let them participate in your care, such as, by inserting a test strip into the blood glucose machine and guessing what your number will be."[4]

Dates, Boyfriends, Partners, and Others:
Diabetes is easy to hide and many women will hold off on sharing the information with a romantic partner for fear of rejection.

- Tell your date/boyfriend when you are ready; don't feel like you have to share this personal information right away.
- Remember that being honest can foster intimacy.

Heather Jacobs says that her experience in sharing the news of her diagnosis with classmates in third grade was not a success:

After spending a couple of weeks in the hospital and some time at home adjusting, I was allowed to return to school. My teacher asked me if I would share my experience with my class, which I did happily. I even brought props! I told my classmates what happened, what I knew about diabetes (basically, I wasn't allowed to eat sugar and I had to take insulin shots), and demonstrated how to draw up insulin, hence the props. I realized by recess that my classmates did not receive the information well, as I was treated like I had the worst case of "cooties" ever to hit Mission Elementary. The children did not want to touch me, drink out of the water fountain after me, because they were afraid they would "catch diabetes" and would have to take shots and not be allowed to eat candy. It really traumatized me and taught me a lesson that took years to unlearn. Fortunately, I moved A LOT and ended up in a new town and new school less than a year later, but I never forgot what I learned.

Heather says having diabetes taught her to lie and how to show people what they wanted to see while doing as she pleased. She says that she now has a much different view of diabetes that she shares with others:

In my opinion, I may not have power over diabetes, but I do have influence over how diabetes affects my life. Today, I cherish my ability to influence this aspect of my life. This influence is panning out in my life, as I have lived with diabetes for nearly 32 years and have reversed many of my complications associated with my years of trying to die young. For the record, I turned 40 this past year and can honestly say that I am living well with diabetes!

Lesley Hoffman Goldenberg was overwhelmed with the positive reaction she received from family and friends:

My family and friends were amazingly supportive. People cooked healthy dinners for my family and dropped them off, my friends wanted to learn everything about diabetes so they could help me, neighbors brought over a bouquet of sugar-free candy because they knew I could eat that. For the most part, friends and family were supportive, curious, and wonderful. However, I do remember once in seventh grade, one of my friends accidentally touched my blood monitor—not the needle part—but the actual monitor. Her mom called my mom the next day to see how I was feeling and doing and just to chat. Somewhere in the conversation, she worked in that her daughter (my friend) had accidentally touched my blood sugar monitor and asked if diabetes was contagious and if her daughter was now at risk. My mom patiently told her that her daughter would be fine and handled it very well—but we still make fun of her for asking that question and it's 16 years later!

A major factor in creating a foundation of understanding and acceptance of diabetes in oneself and in others can depend on the way a woman's diagnosis is managed from the beginning. Meeting with a team of professionals that includes an endocrinologist, a nutritionist, a therapist, and an educator will allow for the greatest success in managing and taking responsibility of the disease.

FINDING THE RIGHT MEDICAL TEAM

After graduating from college, I drove across the country from Colorado to South Carolina where my mom had recently moved with my stepfather. Up until that time, I'd been working with my pediatrician, the same doctor who diagnosed me at 14 years old. After a dismal appointment with an endocrinologist in South Carolina (the doctor's waiting room was filled with old, very sick-looking people and the female doctor was way too perky for my taste), a family friend gave my mom the name of another endocrinologist in Charleston where we lived. I loved Dr. Colwell from the first visit. He was an older man with white hair and a warm smile. He was also involved in the Diabetes Control and Complications Trial (DCCT) research and had started a multidisciplinary team approach to living with diabetes called the Intensive Diabetes Education and Awareness Lifestyle (IDEAL) program. I hadn't been taking care of myself for years, but with his nonjudgmental and warm, intelligent manner, Dr. Colwell got me started on the right track. He was my doctor for more than 10 years, supporting me through some bad low blood sugar episodes and two of my three pregnancies.

When he retired several years ago, I was lost. Who would I see, and where would I go? I didn't want to start all over with someone new. Dr. Colwell knew everything about me, I didn't have to explain to him about the ridiculous notion of counting carbs, he knew that I took care of myself and gave me all kinds of kudos for my good A1cs. Thankfully, I used my contacts and was able to find another wonderful doctor. She was even able to steer me toward the insulin pump, something I'd refused with Dr. Colwell.

Women with diabetes need specialized care, and because living with diabetes is like a full-time job, we need a solid team of medical professionals as a support system. Many studies show that the best way to stay healthy is with the support of a team that includes a doctor, an educator, a nutritionist, and a therapist. However, there are currently about 3,000 endocrinologists and about 25 million people with diabetes in the United States, and of the 3,000 endocrinologists, only about half specialize in diabetes care.

TIPS ON FINDING THE RIGHT DOCTOR

■ Search websites and blogs from fellow people with diabetes in your area and ask who they recommend.
■ Look at the ADA provider listings to find a physician who has met the criteria of the ADA's Provider Recognition Program.
■ Call (800) TEAMUP4, a service of the American Association of Diabetes Educators. They have listings of doctors who are diabetes educators, as well as diabetes nurses and other health professionals who can help you find an appropriate diabetes doctor.
■ Search for a diabetes support group and ask the members for referrals.

Many women are natural people pleasers, which can set up an unequal relationship with the doctor. We can be too concerned with getting a virtual pat on the head for a good A1c and avoid discussing the frequent highs or lows. With the numbers, highs and lows, and patient responsibility, diabetes can create a "good girl, bad girl" pattern. When our blood sugar is high, we are the ones to blame. When it gets low, it's because we gave ourselves too much insulin or didn't eat enough lunch; the responsibility falls largely on our shoulders, which can result in frustration and self-blame. That's one of the reasons why it's so important to not only find a good doctor, whether it's an endocrinologist or a general practitioner, but also a therapist, a nutritionist, and an educator.

MEETING WITH THE DOCTOR/MAKING THE MOST OF YOUR APPOINTMENTS

■ Be proactive, take an active role in management.
■ Go to your doctor prepared with specific questions.
■ Be realistic; set attainable behavioral goals for yourself.

Andi Kravitz Weiss, MPH, a behaviorist at MicroMass Communications in North Carolina, says:

> *It's important for women with diabetes to feel invested in their treatment plan. They should feel empowered to talk to their doctor about which specific aspects of their diabetes they want to focus on. This also means choosing a doctor who values partnering with patients in this capacity. When women work with their doctors to set tangible and achievable treatment goals they feel good about, they are more likely to reach them and have better health outcomes.*

QUESTIONS AND ANSWERS WITH ELIZABETH STEPHENS AND LYNDSAY RIFFE

Why me? How did I get this?

"After a new diagnosis, people often have a lot of guilt, and think that getting diabetes could have been avoided. Explaining what diabetes is, as well as risk factors, (genetics, age, weight, ethnicity) is discussed to try to lift that guilt, as well as encourage," Lyndsay Riffe says.

"I help answer those questions with antibody testing because many of my patients can't get past the 'why me' stage until they have all the information," Dr. Stephens says. She adds, "I try to customize my visits to the individual. It's important to let them know what's practical and realistic."

"Just like diabetes treatment is not one size fits all, so is the approach I take as a diabetes educator when someone is newly diagnosed. Some like to know very basic information after being diagnosed, where others try to get as much information as possible. I understand how the information can be very overwhelming, and try not to overload someone with too much immediately . . . . After being diagnosed with diabetes, patients, generally, have a lot of questions. Time is spent answering questions, and making sure when they leave [the office] that they have a clear understanding of how to take medications, and what to do if a hypoglycemic event occurs (survival skills)," says Lyndsay Riffe.

Can I have children?

Dr. Stephens says that having diabetes is a powerful tool because with two children of her own, she can use herself as a model. "I tell my patients that it comes down to you as a person with diabetes, I give them information and explain that I've done well because I've taken care of myself."

Will I still be able to eat hot fudge sundaes and Cherry Coke?

"With an initial diagnosis, I generally discuss how food affects the blood sugar. I prefer that approach rather than using the term "diet." Depending on the individual's base knowledge of nutrition, I try to have them at least understand that it is carbohydrates, not sugar alone that affect blood glucose levels. Although I believe meal planning is the cornerstone of treating any type of diabetes, this is a subject that can get overwhelming; therefore, I try to gauge where the patient is and make appropriate follow-up appointment to focus on nutrition," Lyndsay Riffe says.

"An occasional hot fudge sundae is the key to life," Dr. Stephens says with a smile.

Will I be able to run, do yoga, swim, dance, bike, travel, work, live alone?

Dr. Stephens says, "I bike to work, so again, I think I am a good model for my patients, but I stress that exercise is just another variable." She says that exercise is different for people with type 1 and type 2 diabetes, who often need to get on an exercise regimen to lose weight. She was the first doctor I've spoken to who was honest about exercise and the challenges. Most often, doctors stress the importance of exercise for women with diabetes, and although it is important to a healthy lifestyle, it isn't easy for people with diabetes.

Am I going to die, go blind, have kidney failure, and have amputations?

Fear and depression are common reactions/responses to a diagnosis of diabetes. Dr. Stephens says that counseling and medication are sometimes necessary.

Develop Your Personal Diabetes Philosophy

Dr. Ann Albright PhD, RD, the Director of the Division of Diabetes Translation at the CDC, has had type 1 diabetes for more than 40 years. Developing a "personal philosophy" was a key factor in managing her diabetes. Dr. Albright's philosophy was influenced by her mother, a nurse, who encouraged Ann to experience life to the fullest. "Diabetes will not define you but is an important part of who you are. It's a philosophy that will serve you well."

Dr. Albright says coping strategies are an important factor toward adjustment and that more and more clinicians are talking about coping skills with people with diabetes. "It's important to come to the starting gate with a willingness to address problems," she says. "It's also important to find balance in how you manage the responsibilities of diabetes and how you live life fully."

Dr. Albright suggests:

- Getting involved with organizations that serve people with diabetes, such as the ADA and the Juvenile Diabetes Research Foundation.
- Give back, raise and/or donate money and/or time to diabetes organizations.
- Contribute to the support system—ask not just what can I get but what can I give? It's empowering to give back and contribute.
- Find healthy venues for expression because "we all have challenging days."

Judith Jones Ambrosini has come a long way from the early days of her diagnosis when she wondered, "Why bother living?" For years, she rode a seesaw of uneducated diabetes management:

Sometimes, I carried a little scale in my book bag and weighed carrot and celery sticks. Sometimes I, yes, ate hot fudge sundaes. I became interested in how I could have diabetes and eat wonderful food. I started to cook. After college, I moved to Italy with my husband at the time and with Jude, my infant son. I began the process of eating the freshest purest food that was filled with art and beauty. I exercised vigorously before the word came into popular vocabulary. I walked and hiked and did yoga with a

70-year-old ballerina who lived next door to me in a small village on the Amalfi coast. The insulin regimen was still a lousy shot of NPH daily. Urine tests were all we had then. It really was the stone age of diabetes care. But I got through it, became a chef, a runner, an ADA board member, and in 1988, became fully committed to a wonderful life with diabetes. It continues. I am by nature an over-the-top optimist. If I feel low about something, I go for a walk, a bike ride, or dance around the kitchen. I call a friend I haven't seen in a while. I go out for a nice dinner and a glass of very good red wine. But usually, I wake up in the morning thankful for another day of sunshine or rain.

GENERAL ADVICE TO WOMEN NEWLY DIAGNOSED

- Take it one day at a time. Diabetes is real, don't deny it but learn all that you can.
- Diabetes doesn't mean your life has to be a prison sentence. You can manage the disease and still enjoy your life and be a free spirit!
- Remember that you can still do everything that you have always done, just in a healthier way.
- It really helps to keep a log about your emotions, stress levels, physical state and activity, mental state, anger level, sleep length and quality, in addition to a food log—all of this affects your blood glucose.
- Be inspiring, but don't be a hero. Allow yourself to feel all the emotions without dwelling on what cannot be changed, and find a source of support from those who truly understand.
- Try to find balance between enjoying yourself and looking after your health, which is not always easy.
- Come to terms with blood sugar testing. It will always be necessary for control and it's your most powerful personal tool.

2   Managing Adolescence

Soon after I was diagnosed at 14 years of age, my mom took me to a support group meeting for parents and kids with type 1 diabetes. Sitting in the circle of the hospital's folding chairs, I listened to the stories of mothers who did insulin shots for their kids and who didn't allow their kids to go on sleepovers for fear that they might suddenly get low blood sugar. I had only lived with this disease for a few days, but I couldn't imagine my mom doing my insulin shot for me. I wasn't allowed to leave the hospital until I could do a shot, and from the very first day, I'd been piercing my own skin. My parents told me that diabetes was not going to define me and I believed them. Looking around the room of the support group, the kids seemed passive, and I realized that I was not going to be like them. I was not going to let diabetes keep me from doing anything my friends were doing, and as a teenager, that included driving, dating, drinking, going away to school, and other independence-seeking activities.

Stella Biggs said that when she was first diagnosed with diabetes, most of her friends and family had no idea what it was:

> *Maybe someone had an aunt who died from [diabetes], but it didn't seem to be around as much. I found out when I was 16, and I was mad about having to change my life-style, along with all the other pressures of being a teenager. I didn't tell everyone. I think I was in denial for a long time. I still wanted to be able to go to Dairy Queen with my friends and eat a Blizzard after school. My immediate friends found out, but I did not tell everyone I knew, and I was taking shots, so it wasn't like they could see the pump on me. I also wasn't testing as much as I should, so most did not know. My biggest frustration as a teenager was not*

being able to act what I thought was normal. I now see that was not true and insignificant, but to a teenager, "fitting in" is up on the list. I don't think I was depressed, I was just in denial a lot of the time. I did not have much control over my diabetes, and had no idea what low blood sugar was, because mine was usually high. I talked to my mother, because she had polio as a child, which is much worse than my diabetes, but she knew how to handle the difficulties of "being different." Again, I don't think it would be quite as hard now as a teenager, with all the availability of sugar substitutes that taste great, but even now, most teenagers don't want to be different than everyone else.

STATISTICS

- Diabetes is one of the most common diseases in adolescence. According to the National Diabetes Fact Sheet, about 215,000 young people in the United States under age 20 had diabetes in 2010. This represents 0.26 percent of all people in this age group.
- Type 2 diabetes is rare in children younger than 10 years of age, regardless of race or ethnicity. After 10 years of age, type 2 diabetes becomes increasingly common, especially in minority populations, representing 14.9 percent of newly diagnosed cases of diabetes in non-Hispanic whites, 46.1 percent in Hispanic youth, 57.8 percent in African Americans, 69.7 percent in Asian/ Pacific Islanders, and 86.2 percent in American Indian youth.

Source: Centers for Disease Control and Prevention (CDC).

Kayla is a teenager at Goose Creek, South Carolina. She is pretty, with long, blonde hair and is a cheerleader. She lives at home with her parents and younger sister. She has everything going for her, *and* she has diabetes.

"No one knows what it's like to have diabetes," Kayla says. There are other kids at her school with diabetes, but they are not her friends. She goes to Camp Adam Fisher every summer where she connects with other kids with diabetes, but that is only 1 week each year. Kayla has a photo album filled with pictures of her and other young girls in bikinis at the lake with their arms around each other. If you look close, you can see a pump on several of the young women.

At 16 years old, Kayla is seeing a psychiatrist for adherence issues. About a year ago, she started trying to ignore her diabetes. With a far off smile she said:

> *I didn't want to deal with it or have the responsibility anymore. I got tired of it and I want more than anything for it to just go away. Now, I'm at the point where I have completely shut it out of my life. I hardly ever check my blood sugars, take insulin, or change my sites. It's past the point of "ignoring" it, and I think it's more that I have completely forgotten about it. When I sit down to eat, the need to check my blood sugar or take insulin doesn't even cross my mind. Before, I used to brush it off and say, "Oh well!" But now, I don't even remember. I've gotten rid of it in a way.*

She adds:

> *Diabetes upsets me for many different reasons. I wish I could be like everyone else and not worry about checking my blood sugar, taking insulin, remembering to pack and bring extra supplies everywhere, count my carbs at every meal, or change my pump sites. I'm a teenager, and all this extra "stuff" makes me feel very overwhelmed.*

Kayla says she can remember what it was like before she was diagnosed. Everything was easier and "more fun." She worries that teachers and coaches think she's using diabetes as an excuse to get out of doing stuff, "but that's not it at all." Kayla feels like diabetes gets in the way of everything, "like an annoying little bug that flies around your head, and as much as you try to swat at it, it won't go away."

Sloan Wesloh says:

> *When I went to public high school, I was the only one in the entire school with diabetes. I went back to school 2 days after coming home from the hospital where I was diagnosed with diabetes. I didn't know anyone with*

*diabetes; people were asking me why I had diabetes
when I wasn't obese, and I had to go to the principal's
office to meet my mom to take a shot at lunch. I felt so
incredibly alone.*

SELF-ESTEEM

Studies show that teens with a vulnerable sense of self may struggle to
manage the complex demands of diabetes. A negative or positive self-
concept can predict metabolic control in adolescent girls.

In the article "Metabolic Control in Adolescent Girls: Links to Relationality and the Female Sense of Self," Maharaj et al. state:

> *Positive perceptions of one's behavioral conduct (i.e., the
> ability to act the way one is supposed to and avoid "get-
> ting into trouble") was associated with lower HbA1c levels.
> Achieving and maintaining good metabolic control
> requires adherence to a complex, multi-component treat-
> ment regimen that is difficult for many teens to master.
> These difficulties may further contribute to heightened
> feelings of helplessness and ineffectiveness. Thus, a positive
> self-concept may be an important developmental buffer
> that promotes successful adaptation among adolescent
> girls with diabetes who face concomitant stresses associ-
> ated with the demands of a chronic illness and the devel-
> opmental transitions of adolescence.*[1]

Mallory Boyd was diagnosed at 9 years old and says that as a middle
child, she fits the classic definition of independent, middle child behavior:

> *I have really always been independent. Even with my
> diabetes I chose to talk with others about my experi-
> ences and how they can also live a normal life. It was
> difficult at times to explain to my parents why I didn't
> like their involvement in monitoring my sugar levels.
> However, I think their constant worry and checking
> helped me to develop a better sense of how to control
> my diabetes.*

*I am always in need of improvement, but having my
parents attend pump education classes and nutritional
classes helped me feel more connected with the struggles of
having diabetes.*

*I did feel like my parents kept a tight control on how I
handled my diabetes, but never to an extent that I
resented them. Because of my diabetes, I felt I matured a
lot faster and was given more opportunities to act older.
My parents trusted me because I think they knew I would
never drink because of my diabetes, and therefore, I was
allowed to stay out later than many of my friends.*

SOCIAL ACCEPTANCE

The "Metabolic Control in Adolescent Girls" study showed that social acceptance among girls is associated with higher hemoglobin A1c (HbA1c). That
is, girls who are not making diabetes management a priority have more
friends but are sacrificing a low A1c.

*Striving for social acceptance may be problematic for girls
with a chronic medical illness such as diabetes, which makes
them feel "different" from their nondiabetic peers. Vulnerable girls who seek social acceptance and connection may be
more likely to conform to social pressures [and] to engage in
behaviors that may adversely impact metabolic control.[1]*

Cheryl Alkon, who was diagnosed as a child, didn't worry about fitting in:

*When I was maybe 12 or 13, I went to a party my swim
team was having, and I remember one of the coaches went
out of her way to empty out a can of non-diet root beer and
pour my Diet Coke into it so that I wouldn't look different
than the other kids who were drinking root beer and other
regular soda at the party. I remember thinking that she
didn't have to do that, that I'd been used to drinking my diet
soda at parties for a while, and that I'd been fine with it.*

Heather Jacobs kept her diabetes a secret from her friends. After going into a coma when she was diagnosed, her pediatrician gave her parents the advice to not allow diabetes to be an excuse from living life. Heather says that her parents took the pediatrician's advice to mean, "Don't talk about Heather's diabetes."

> *I learned in third grade that I was better off keeping knowledge of my diabetes to myself. We lived "as if" I didn't have diabetes and rarely ever talked about it, other than my blood sugars . . . . Given my early experiences and awkward family dynamics, I chose to refrain from telling people that I lived with diabetes. I lived in the closet with my diabetes for over a decade. I did a phenomenal job of hiding my diabetes over my school years. No one knew, including my closest high school friends, about my condition, that is until I was accidentally "outed" by my dad. When I was 17, I got really sick with bronchitis and out-of-control blood sugars and landed myself in the ICU. My dad openly discussed my situation with his business partner, who happened to be the dad of two kids in my class. By the time I got back to school, it seemed like everyone knew about my secret. I felt shamed, embarrassed, judged, and violated. My cover was blown. I could no longer do as I pleased without someone telling me, "You can't eat that." My close friends were shocked and amazed that I had diabetes and that I didn't tell them. It wasn't very difficult to hide, especially since I rarely tested my glucose, and when I needed to take my shot, I would simply go to the bathroom. I thought I was so sly.*

INDEPENDENCE

A young woman's relationship with her parents is of great importance during this stage of life.

Tim Wysocki, writing in the journal *Diabetes Spectrum*, says:

> *Pushing adolescents too hard toward autonomy in self-care may actually impede their internalization of positive health values. We know that teenagers who assume*

diabetes responsibilities too soon face increased risks of
problems with treatment adherence, poor diabetic control,
and preventable hospitalizations.[2]

Cheryl Alkon's mother was very involved with her diabetes when
she was diagnosed:

> *Throughout my childhood, and when I was looking at*
> *colleges, she urged me to choose more local colleges (i.e.,*
> *closer to New England where I lived, than say, California).*
> *As she put it, "If you're going to get an English degree, why*
> *go all the way across the country for it?" While she didn't*
> *come out and say it, I think she was worried that some-*
> *thing might happen to me with diabetes that may have*
> *been tougher to deal with if I was far away. I did look at*
> *colleges outside of New England, but ultimately applied*
> *to those that were, except for a few, in my home state of*
> *Massachusetts. (To be fair, there are some excellent schools*
> *in Massachusetts.) But yes, I am sure my mother worried*
> *about me far more as I was the older daughter with type 1*
> *than she worried about my younger brother (3 years*
> *younger) who did not have diabetes. I couldn't wait to go*
> *to college and be out from under my parents' eyes, but I*
> *didn't do much crazy stuff once I was there.*

Katie Savin's parents divorced soon after her diagnosis, and when her
older sister went off to college, she found herself largely on her own. "When
I was 16, my parents divorced and my diabetes went out the window." Katie's
dad moved out and her mom was busy with a new job, and with little parental supervision, her house became "party central." Katie maintained the illu-
sion that everything was okay on the outside, but on the inside, she was
skipping injections, drinking, and rebelling against the control of diabetes.

Lesley Hoffman Goldenberg felt like her parents gave her a lot of
independence. She had her own car and was allowed to drive wherever
she wanted:

> *When I went to camp the summer after my freshman year*
> *of college, my parents realized my diabetes was totally out*
> *of control and something needed to be done. My mom*
> *wrote me a letter at camp and she basically said, "I see*

*how difficult diabetes is. I would take on diabetes for you
if it meant that you didn't have it, but that's not possible.
You need to start checking your blood sugar, get your A1c
down, eat right, and exercise, otherwise, I'm pulling you
out of college and you're moving back to the Midwest and
living at home, under our control."*

Her mother's warning motivated Lesley to get herself back on track
so she could maintain her independence.

Maia Caemmerer was diagnosed right as she was leaving for college:

*Safe to say, I am in charge of my health and have been
from day one. I know, without any uncertainty, that I
know so much more about my body, my health, and my
responsibility to myself than my peers. I am the last call on
keeping myself alive. I am in charge of my ultimate
well-being, and nobody else I know (at my age) realizes
that they, too, are in charge of theirs.*

ACCOMMODATIONS AT SCHOOL

Managing the day-to-day complexities of diabetes at school can be a challenge. Every school is different, and the plan for managing diabetes at school should be customized for each young woman. The Americans with Disabilities Act provides regulations for people with diabetes. Special considerations would include meal planning, blood glucose (BG) testing, and snacks on field trips.

- Set up a meeting with teachers/administrators/nurse/counselor/coach to write a diabetes medical management plan (DMMP) for BG testing; eating requirements; and unusual circumstances such as field trips, sports events, and so forth. (Sample plans can be found at the American Diabetes Association [ADA] website: http://www.diabetes.org/.)
- Write up a 504 plan. This document takes the information in the DMMP and explains the school's specific responsibilities. It is developed to protect a child's rights under relevant federal laws. One thing the plan addresses is who else should be trained to provide diabetes care tasks for your child when the school nurse is not available.

■ Arrange for a place to keep supplies including sugar for lows.

■ Talk to friends and classmates.

■ Request accommodations during standardized testing sessions from testing agencies (such as sugar, monitor, and breaks). You may have to provide a letter from a doctor or an individualized educational plan (IEP) if you have one. To request for accommodations, you may contact the following testing agencies: *International Baccalaureate* at (212) 696-4464; *ACT Services for Students with Disabilities* at (319) 337-1000; or the *College Board Services for Students with Disabilities* at (609) 771-7137.

I went to the University of Colorado in Boulder, a school with more than 30,000 students. I remember walking into my first class—it was a required lecture class with 500 students—and realized that no one would even know I was there. I was not proactive about asking for any kind of accommodations for my diabetes, because I was still in denial and more concerned with fitting in than standing out. I didn't want to ask for extra help. Looking back, I realize how much I could have benefited in high school and college if I had asked for breaks during tests to check my blood sugar. But the last thing I wanted was to be singled out. Although my experience was not the universal experience of women with diabetes, it seems like that the first step toward asking for accommodations at school needs to be the acceptance of the disease. The ADA website provides information about accommodations for college students with diabetes.

Although the precise name will vary, most colleges have an office of disability services that coordinates the disability assistance for students. Information about this office should be available on the college's website, in the official bulletin, or from the registrar or the academic dean. Registering with this office is the first step you should take to put your college on notice of your diabetes and to request modifications on this basis.

Once registered, students can receive modifications through the office, and it can assist students in working with other officials throughout the college. For example, it can help a student on an athletic team solve a dispute with the athletic department or assist a student seeking nutritional information from dining services.

Additionally, many disability services offices provide students with "accommodation letters" to give to their professors at the beginning of every semester. These letters give professors notice that students have registered with the disability services office and have come to an agreement that certain modifications will be provided.

Maia Caemmerer says she let professors know upfront about her diabetes:

> *I didn't tell one professor, and when I grabbed a snack in the middle of an exam she pulled me aside, I told her I was diabetic and she asked to see my state medical card! I told her that if she wanted me to pass out in class and cause an even bigger scene I could do that, too, and that I would call the paramedics in advance next time so they would know to come [and] give me a boost. Safe to say, she lets me eat whenever I need to. Other than that, I've yet to come up against any trouble.*

DRIVING

One of the major health care companies, Medtronic Diabetes, has now come out with a new program to educate teenage drivers who have diabetes. Medtronic Diabetes is the only company that has a U.S. Food and Drug Administration (FDA)-approved integrated insulin pump and continuous glucose monitoring system. The company created a 1-day safe driving course called *Test B4U Drive*, currently held in Colorado, California, Nevada, and Illinois.

"Teenagers with diabetes, like adults, can drive effectively and be safe, but it means developing a plan ahead of time," says Dr. Francine R. Kaufman, chief medical officer and vice president of the Global Medical, Clinical and Health Affairs at Medtronic. "It's critically important for teens with diabetes to manage their glucose levels. A low glucose level can impair judgment, which can be particularly dangerous behind the wheel of a car."

Sloan Wesloh says:

> *In order to get my driver's license, my endocrinologist requires that I have an A1c under 9 percent, I wear a medical alert symbol, and that I check my blood sugar four or more times a day. I worry a lot about getting my license and having the responsibility to drive safely with diabetes. I know of some people who have a general rule*

of testing their blood sugar before getting in their car and only driving when their blood sugar is above, say, 100 mg/dl and below 300 mg/dl (for example). I plan to have something like this set for myself, but I'm not so sure about testing every time I get into the car. That's a lot to ask of a teenager, but I'd like to set it as a goal for myself once I start driving.

TIPS FOR SAFE DRIVING

- If you take insulin, you are at risk for hypoglycemia (low blood sugar reactions) at any time. If this happens when you are driving, you must pull the car over to the side of the road right away and treat your low blood sugar (glucose) reaction. You should always carry rapid-acting carbohydrates (glucose or sugar) and extra snacks to treat any low blood sugar reactions. Keep glucose tablets or other sources of carbohydrates with you and in your car at all times.
- If you have any trouble recognizing your symptoms of low blood sugar (which often happens in people who have very tight BG control), you must check your blood sugar before you start to drive. This is also a good idea for anyone who is going on a long drive. If your blood sugar level is lower than 80 mg/dl, treat it with 10–15 grams of carbohydrate, followed by a snack. This way, you can prevent serious low blood sugar while you are driving.
- It is important that you wear some form of medical identification (bracelet or necklace) to alert others that you have diabetes and use insulin. This could save your life if you have an accident and are unconscious. The medical rescue team will alert others that you have diabetes and may need sugar or insulin.
- Don't leave BG meters, test strips, or insulin in the car. Changes in temperature can damage them.
- Even without symptoms, you should check your BG levels at regular times.[3]

Source: Joslin Diabetes Center.

DRINKING

Drinking is another stage in an adolescent's life that can be further complicated with diabetes.

Lesley Hoffman Goldenberg says that someone along the way scared the wits out of her when it comes to drinking and diabetes, and as a result, she does not drink:

> *I may have a glass of white wine with dinner maybe once every few months but that is it. I can't trace it, but someone must have said something to me and I just can't drink. I'm too scared. I have the most supportive family, amazing friends, and a wonderful fiancé who would never let anything happen to me if I drank and got too low, but I just can't do it. I always say—I'm fun without alcohol, why drink?*

So, is drinking acceptable if you have diabetes? The answer is yes, in moderation, providing that you take the proper precautions. People with diabetes can consume alcohol in moderation. Take into consideration the medication used to control your diabetes and the timing of your meals. Alcohol should be consumed along with a meal or a substantial snack of at least 15 grams of carbohydrates. Drinking alcohol adds extra caloric intake, and drinking calorie-free beverages, especially in addition to alcohol, is best for people with diabetes.

The ADA asserts that alcohol can be incorporated into a diet plan, provided that blood sugar control is already well established and other conditions that aren't compatible with alcohol consumption (such as pregnancy or certain diabetic complications) don't exist.

When you drink, your liver decreases its ability to release glucose so that it can clean the alcohol from your blood. Because glucose production is shut down, hypoglycemia becomes a risk for people with diabetes, particularly if you drink on an empty stomach or shortly after taking insulin or glucose-lowering oral medications. And because it takes 2 hours for just 1 ounce of alcohol to metabolize and leave your system, the risk continues long after you've emptied your glass.

For individuals with well-controlled diabetes, alcohol intake should follow the same guidelines that the U.S. Department of Agriculture (USDA) has established for the general population. This means a maximum of two drinks per day for men and one drink daily for women. (A higher alcohol intake is allowed for most men because women have a lower body water content than men and metabolize alcohol more slowly.) In addition, because of physiological changes such as loss of lean body mass that occur as the body ages, the National Institute on Alcohol Abuse and Alcoholism recommends that anyone older than 65 years old should not consume more than one alcoholic drink daily. One drink is defined as:

- 12 ounces of regular beer (150 calories)
- 5 ounces of wine (100 calories)
- 1.5 ounces of 80-proof distilled spirits (100 calories)

Maia Caemmerer says:

I make it a point to keep my blood sugar around 150 when I am drinking. Alcohol can lower your blood sugar a lot over time, so knowing that you're safe from a sneak-attack low BS in the middle of the night is a good idea. The other thing I do is that I find one person that I trust unconditionally, and explain to them that no matter how drunk I may seem, if I pass out for any reason, to give me my glucagon shot. I show them how to do it, and put it in a safe place with all my other supplies. For me, this is usually my boyfriend or a host of the party I am at. But whoever it may be, having one responsible person who can take care of you in an emergency is a good idea. If it turns out [that] you passed out because you had a few too many beers, then your blood sugar goes up, but it is better safe than sorry.

Avoid dark beers, boxed wine, and high-carb mixers. Low-carb sodas are great as mixers, and light beers are about carb-neutral.

TIPS ABOUT DRINKING AND DIABETES

- Avoid sweet drinks
- Always eat something when drinking
- Always test blood sugar when drinking

Moderate and excessive alcohol consumption affects BG levels, causing hypoglycemia or hyperglycemia. If you drink too much, you may fail to recognize the symptoms of hypoglycemia.

- Always carry sugar in case of low blood sugar

The symptoms of drinking in excess and low glucose levels are similar and very dangerous, especially when taking insulin.

DATING AND SEX

Sexuality is another adolescent stepping stone, and the ways in which it relates to diabetes may seem less clear. However, having sex, whether it's the first time or not, is a physical act. Diabetes is a disease of the body, and whether a young woman wears an insulin pump or bears the scars of finger testing or lumps and bruises from years of injections, diabetes is a visibly physical disease. (We will discuss this topic in more depth in Chapter 6.) What matters is that adolescents need to feel comfortable with their bodies so they can tell the person they are dating about them having diabetes and not feel ashamed. Confidence will also enable teens to ask questions to their doctors, parents, and friends when needed.

Sloan Wesloh says:

> *To me, I feel more attractive when I am able to walk confidently with my pump on my side and people knowing that I have diabetes, but I don't let it get me down. I feel that the right guy for me will like me being confident and not self-conscious about my diabetes. Of course, diabetes does make it hard sometimes to feel beautiful. Sometimes, I hate how my pump or my blood-stained fingers look.*

This summer I refrained from buying that super cute bikini swimsuit because of the pump marks on my stomach that make me feel gross. But this summer I also attended diabetes camp, where everyone has diabetes. At the beach I was with other girls who had the same scars and who were not self-conscious at all about them. That made me realize that being that way—being who you are—makes you truly beautiful.

Stella Biggs says:

Depending on how serious I was with my date, I only told about my diabetes, at first, if we were in an eating situation. As things progressed and got more serious, I obviously had to tell everything. Most of the guys I dated did not know much about diabetes, so I told them what I knew and how it affected me and them and what to expect. I was a little self-conscious about carrying syringes around. I didn't want anyone to think I was a drug addict, because it wasn't as common as it is now, in my opinion. Being a diabetic did not affect my feelings of attractiveness. Being a teenager, I was not concerned that guys would see me differently, although I didn't explain everything right away to them. My choices about sexual behavior had nothing to do with being diabetic at all. I was not a sexually active teen, due to my own personal choices, which had nothing to do with having diabetes.

Kristin Makszin thinks it is incredibly important to bring up diabetes with people you date to see how they react:

The truth is that you need someone who is understanding and supportive. When my husband and I started dating, I was pretty open with him about diabetes. He says that he felt really honored that I was willing to share with him personal stuff when we had only been on a few dates. And then he began learning. Now he knows almost everything about diabetes. I can tell him the blood sugar number and he knows what to do. But he has learned from me and still

*trusts that I know what is best for me. So he is a support
for my diabetes, but not the boss of my diabetes. I think
that it is a delicate but important balance.*

*He does ask questions sometimes, like if it is good that
I am eating this or doing that, but it is just him trying to
understand. And if it is actually not a good idea, then
I realize it, too!*

*I think that diabetes can be a good way to make sure that
you find a caring person, which you want anyway. So
I highly recommend being open about your diabetes when
you are ready. If it's the right person, they will care and
want to learn about you and your diabetes.*

The Centers for Disease Control and Prevention (CDC) report, *Diabetes and Women's Health Across the Life Stages*, states that the appropriate time to begin discussions about responsible family planning and the impact of diabetes on pregnancy and childbearing is during the middle school years as adolescent girls mature. This discussion can be positive, emphasizing the likelihood of a future normal pregnancy and of the birth of a healthy baby, if careful attention is paid to diabetes control prior to and throughout the pregnancy and delivery. It is helpful for the adolescent and her parents to hear this discussion because popular culture often presents childbearing in a woman with diabetes as being difficult or impossible.

For the teen who chooses to be sexually active, confidential counseling on appropriate birth control or referral for these services should be part of the diabetes health care team's routine practice. The importance of preconception counseling cannot be overemphasized to the teen, as well as the need for early notification of the diabetes health care team when an unplanned pregnancy is suspected. The risk of congenital anomalies in the offspring is reduced tenfold by careful diabetes management in the 3 months prior to and during pregnancy. The care of the pregnant patient with diabetes is one of the major recent advances in diabetes care, and the adolescent patient should be made aware of the importance of intensified diabetes management during this time of her life so she and her unborn child can benefit from this new information.

Dr. Albright says a typical concern for teens is whether anyone will find them attractive. "A lot of that anchors back to the ability that you've had over time to develop a philosophy about how you live with diabetes."

She continues:

> *A lot of your feelings are going to be shaped and formed by when you were diagnosed with diabetes and what experiences you had when you developed diabetes. That will affect whether you develop a healthy outlook. And of course, when you hit the teen and adolescent years, my friend and colleague Dr. Fran Kauffman says you have two diseases, diabetes and adolescence. You're dealing with a lot of turmoil during those years, sexual issues, possibly drugs and alcohol, eating disorders, but it's been my observation that the reaction to those issues is most anchored in your coping capabilities. It isn't enough with diabetes to learn about your meds, necessary tests, and exams. You really have got to have guidance and support from family and health care professionals about coping and support.*

Maia Caemmerer started her period a week before she was diagnosed:

> *I was actually diagnosed the week before I started my period, and it shot my BG through the roof. It made for an early diagnosis, that's for sure. As I became more attuned to my blood glucose, I realized that they became incredibly irregular the week before I started my period, with no pattern, rhyme, or reason. I chose to get a Mirena (hormone) IUD. The consistent release of hormones evened out my blood glucose. It was one of the best choices I made for my diabetes, and it took one thing off of my daily health-related to-do list: no more birth control pills!*

PUBERTY

Women with type 1 diabetes were shown to have more menstrual problems (long cycles, long menstruation, and heavy menstruation) before the age of 30 than their nondiabetic peers. Menstrual disorders include late onset, lengthy duration, and heaviness. These disorders can lead to increased risk of osteoporosis and cardiovascular disease. Women with type 1 diabetes experienced menarche nearly a year later than their non-diabetic sisters and control subjects.

In particular, self-report of any menstrual problem, defined as menstrual irregularity or a heavy menstruation, was higher among women with diabetes than their nondiabetic sisters and control subjects for age ranges.

Several authors have also reported a 1-year delay in menarche with type 1 diabetes as well as a later menarche among those with an earlier age at onset. Diabetes onset before puberty may cause weight loss, decreasing the body fat that is important for menarche to occur.

Katie Savin didn't get her period until she was 17 years old. She remembers going to her gynecologist when she was 16, and being told if nothing happened in the next year, then they would be concerned. She got her period before the year was up and didn't worry. However, her period was never regular.

Usually, a woman's insulin requirement goes up 10–15 percent during the last 3–5 days of the menstrual cycle because of the hormone progesterone. This is the hormone that prepares the uterus to be full of extra tissue and blood to receive the egg if it is fertilized. Rising levels of progesterone counteract that action of insulin. During these days, bedtime insulin doses may need to be increased, and possibly, morning insulin doses as well.

The only way to manage changing insulin requirements right before your period is to measure your BG often. Your doctor can help you to figure out what insulin dose adjustments you should make each month before your period.

Stella Biggs says:

I had already started my period before I got diabetes. My cycle was never the same. Sometimes, it lasted 5 days, sometimes 7–8 days, and the flow was inconsistent during my adolescence. I don't remember any changes in the blood sugar levels during menstruation. One thing I did find out, though, was that when I was not taking care of myself at college I did not have my period the whole year, which was great (thank goodness, I wasn't sleeping around or I could have been taking pregnancy tests a lot!). I didn't realize that my blood sugar levels would affect my period.

EMOTIONS

Lesley Hoffman Goldenberg remembers feeling frustrated because she couldn't accomplish a tight diabetes control herself:

My parents were always giving advice or my doctors or other nurses/doctors I encountered at camp. Everyone had their idea of how I could best manage my diabetes and keep my sugars in control. It was frustrating because none of these people actually had diabetes, and none of them were with me all year round—so they didn't know my schedule and how hard I was really trying.

Cheryl Alkon says diabetes didn't play as huge a role in her teenage years. She had other things to worry about, such as:

How to get top grades in school, how to get into the college of my choice, and just balancing my life as a student between studying, things like swim team and yearbook, and my temple youth group. I did a lot of stuff in high school and don't remember much that diabetes stood out. I would just tell people, "You put on deodorant every day. You brush your teeth." I take a shot. It's just something I do.

FAMILY DYNAMICS

Managing diabetes in children and adolescents is most effective when the entire family gets involved. Parents should be alert for signs of depression, eating disorders, or insulin omission to lose weight and seek appropriate treatment. Positive outcomes are more likely for teens who grow up in family and health care environments that have the following characteristics:

- Diabetes management is seen as a vehicle to accomplish broad life goals, rather than being defined more narrowly.
- Loved ones' concerns are expressed through warmth and empathy, and the adolescents become comfortable with relying on the support of others. There is more praise and admiration for self-care success and effort than there is criticism and punishment for self-care failures.

- Diabetes responsibilities are transferred actively to the adolescents for the right reasons rather than as a result of parental burnout.
- Parent–adolescent communication is frequent, mutually respectful, and constructive rather than conflictual and destructive.

Tim Wysocki says:

> *Health care professionals should routinely evaluate families along these dimensions before and after their children with diabetes enter adolescence. Families with significant problems on any of these dimensions should be referred for evaluation and possible treatment by a mental health professional who is familiar with diabetes.*[2]

Sloan Wesloh says that she feels like she has a closer relationship with her parents than most kids do:

> *My parents give me the right amount of independence with diabetes, and I take the responsibility of taking care of myself. My parents are also good about communicating with me when I'm with friends or somewhere and they need to know my "diabetes status" (blood sugars, insulin dosages, etc.) and I don't really want to have a long phone conversation in front of my friends. We text message each other all the time!*
>
> *Having diabetes does have a toll on my family, though. When I am having a high blood sugar (and occasionally, this will happen with low blood sugars, too) I am very cranky. I am not all [sic] there at all and I say (or yell) things that I do not mean. Oftentimes, I don't even remember what I said later. It's hard for my family to understand that I'm not there—it's my blood sugar that is saying those weird things!*

SUMMER CAMPS

One place where the feelings of isolation are eliminated is at summer camps. These camps help kids with diabetes fit in. This need becomes more powerful as children enter adolescence, when they most certainly do not want to stand out in any way. Being surrounded by people who are just like them relaxes the tension that kids feel when they are different. For instance, approximately 80 percent of campers are on insulin pumps. What a relief this can be for a child who usually must explain his or her pump to everyone he or she meets.

In addition to the psychological advantages that camping bestows, real statistics underscore the benefits of camp on the health of young campers. The Joslin Diabetes Center, a teaching and research affiliate of Harvard Medical School, sponsored a study of how diabetes camp affected A1c. Although 1 year of camp had a minimal effect, attending camp for 2, 3, and 4 years caused A1c to drop dramatically.

Unfortunately, only 25 percent of children with type 1 diabetes go to camp. Many children are on waiting lists. There are far too few endocrinologists, diabetes educators, and physicians to staff enough camps for everyone who wants to attend. Only 144 camps serve the entire United States, and some of those are day camps. Only about five or so of the camps are year-around, self-owned facilities.

Sloan Wesloh goes to Camp Needlepoint in Hudson, Wisconsin:

> *I've only gone [to camp] for 2 years; I say **only** 2 years because lots of my camp friends have gone for 10 years or more. I was skeptical about camp at first. People, who aren't close friends of mine, who find out that I'm going to diabetes camp, sometimes think that diabetes camp is either a therapy camp for kids with diabetes or a camp where we learn about eating right and where to do our injections. It's not that at all! At diabetes camp, we don't spend any time learning about diabetes or diets. Instead, we just enjoy our time being normal teenagers with diabetes.*

> *I've been doing the rock-climbing program since I started going to camp. This past year, we went on a trip to Taylors Falls to do some outdoor climbing along the St. Croix River. That was amazing!*

> *It is a different world at camp, and my friends and I look forward to that week, all year long. Camp was the first place most of us got to meet another diabetic kid. It was*

the first place where we learned that there were other kids out there dealing with situations that we thought we were alone in.

I think the most rewarding part about camp is how everyone understands. We know how it feels. Suddenly, you don't have to be so self-conscious about anything, those tape marks on your stomach, giving a shot at dinner, or waking up in the middle of the night for a low. We've all been there. It may seem crazy to say that I love going to a camp where we all test our blood sugar together and compare insulin pumps, but I do and a lot of other kids and teenagers do.

THE TESTING LIMITS PROGRAM

Insulin Independence, an organization for youths with type 1 diabetes, has a program called Testing Limits. This program teaches children and teens that there are no limits to a life with diabetes, and demonstrates how exercise plays a vital role in one's health. Program participants are taught to understand the process of goal setting and the expansion of one's own mental and physical abilities. During the months prior to a Testing Limits Youth Expedition, children or teens with diabetes are paired with type 1 staff mentors, who help the youths prepare for their forthcoming adventure. Once the trip begins, youths are encouraged to rely on one another for support as they confront new challenges despite their diabetes.

Advice from Leslie Goldenberg:

Pick your battles. You won't be in perfect control, and you won't eat perfectly, and your A1c may not be wonderful. Pick a couple of things to focus on and don't get too stressed out. Teenagers have enough to worry about— spend as much time thinking about boys and school dances as you do about insulin and blood sugars (okay, maybe slightly more on diabetes but still). Don't get into the routine of drinking. I have a glass of wine once in a while now that I'm an adult but that's it. I just stayed away from it in high school and because of that, it never became a part of my routine. Try to have your diabetes become a normal part of your group of friends, but not an overwhelming part. No teenager (you, the diabetic, especially) wants to worry about their health, blood sugars, emergencies, etc. at such a young age. Make your friends aware, let them know what needs to be done if you're low ("buy me a Coke!") or if you have a high blood sugar ("get me some water and take me to a toilet"), but don't overwhelm them with information. Good friends will want to learn more, eventually.

3   Diet

When I was diagnosed with type 1 diabetes, one of my first concerns was whether I could still drink Cherry Coke. In 1985, the flavor "cherry" was a recent addition to Coca-Cola products, and there would be no Diet Cherry Coke. My doctor said that whenever I am thirsty, I could drink water, diet soda, or tea; and whenever I am hungry, I could snack on peanuts and pickles—"free foods." These were foods I could eat without giving myself an injection. But I hated pickles and peanuts. I wanted Cherry Coke, not tea.

At 14 years old, I'd only just begun drinking soda. My parents were vegetarian hippies who composted our leftovers and picked fiddleheads from neighboring fields for dinner. They would get our milk from the farm at the end of our dirt road in the woods of a small town in Vermont. Away from my family, at a fancy, private boarding school, I'd been thrilled with the freedom to eat as I pleased for the first time in my life. For the 6 weeks I was at school, I bought sodas from the mini-mart across the street, ate ice cream from the dining hall and cheese steaks and fries from the den. I indulged in all the sugary, sensory delights that I'd been deprived of for my entire childhood, and then, I started being thirsty all the time and falling asleep in class, and after losing 15 pounds in less than a week, I was diagnosed with type 1 diabetes, just like my younger sister.

After my diagnosis, mealtime became a science class with a language of its own: *exchanges*, *starches*, *carbohydrates*, and *simple sugars*. Suddenly, I was supposed to count and measure my food, and before each meal, I had to stick a needle into my skin. If I screwed up and gave myself too much insulin (if I miscalculated the carb to insulin ratio), I would become dizzy and with shaky hands. I had to unwrap yellow, pink, and orange pieces of candy, popping them into my mouth to raise my sugar levels. I had to do this whether I was hungry or not. If I gave myself too

55

little insulin, or was still hungry after my balanced meal and ate a piece of the delicious warm bread that everyone else was eating, then I would pay for its consequences. I would feel bad, sleepy, and thirsty, and would mentally beat myself up for being too greedy and not being a "good diabetic."

For a few weeks, the changes were fun. I enjoyed the times I got low and needed to eat sugar. When I started to feel funny, I was happy because I got to eat the food I was denied on a daily basis. I was told that I could no longer eat certain foods (Cherry Coke, milkshakes, fries, etc.) when I wanted to, but I *had* to eat them when my blood sugar was low. So getting low was fun, because I got to eat the stuff my friends were eating. I was being rewarded for poor management. I felt like a kid in *Charlie and the Chocolate Factory* who wasn't allowed to eat anything, neither the chocolate river, nor the lollipops hanging from the trees, nor the bubblegum flowers; nothing, unless my blood sugar was low.

But after a while, unwrapping the candy with shaky hands and then eating it, sometimes right after I'd finished a big meal, made me feel bad. Why did I have to eat if I wasn't hungry? I felt ashamed of the way my body was unable to regulate itself and was embarrassed to be discovered snacking on Lorna Doone cookies in my bed during study hall, whereas my friends wavered between grapefruit-only diets and, after study hall, pizza binges. My friends could deny and indulge themselves at their whim, whereas I had to plan my meals. I had to carry snacks around with me at all times, and eat on a schedule. I was dependent on food.

HISTORY

The history of a diabetic diet is rooted in carbohydrate restriction. Before Banting and Best discovered insulin in the 1920s, some doctors were keeping people with diabetes alive through drastic measures such as starvation diets. When a patient began to show signs of diabetes, they were put on a "starvation diet." In the book, *The Discovery of Insulin*, author Michael Bliss explains that in 1913, the starvation method was advanced under the direction of Dr. Frederick Allen, a researcher of sugar consumption at Harvard Medical School. Dr. Allen's work deepened the understanding of restricted eating and he decided that, "if over-nourishment or normal nourishment produced diabetic symptoms, then the trick was to find the degree of under-nourishment that would enable a diabetic to live sugar- and symptom-free." Dr. Allen's work was controversial, because he advocated restricting eating at a time when being well-fed was a sign of good health. He was asking patients who came to him complaining of weight loss, insatiable hunger, and thirst, to further restrict their diet. However, his method was one of the only options available and he was keeping people alive. In Bliss's book, Dr. Allen is quoted:

> *In those situations where the awful choice between death from diabetes and death from starvation could not be avoided, comparative observations of patients dying under extreme inanition (starvation) and those dying with active diabetic symptoms produced by lax diets or by violations of diet have convinced us that suffering is distinctly less under the former program.*[1]

The black-and-white photos in books about the history of diabetes show what it looked like to starve to death. There is a photograph of a mother holding her son who is starving, his arms circles her neck, and she holds him up under his bottom for the picture. His face looks like he is filled with pain and he appears to be crying, and the mother's eyes are huge, her mouth is set, and she stares out at the camera. The picture was taken in 1922 and the boy had been living with diabetes for more than 2 years. He looks to be about 5 years old but the book doesn't say so and it's difficult to tell. He was subsisting on a diet of lettuce, broccoli, and cucumbers and his weight at the time of the photograph was 15 pounds. Months after this picture was taken, the unnamed boy was photographed again, after he'd been given insulin. His weight had doubled and he was pictured in a sailor suit, his cheeks were full and he looked like a completely different person. I wish there was a picture of me from when I was sick. I would like to see what a body that was destroyed by its own tissues looked like on me.

One of Dr. Allen's more famous patients was Elizabeth Hughes, the daughter of the secretary of state at the time, Charles Evans Hughes. In 1918, Elizabeth Hughes was 12 years old when she was diagnosed with diabetes. Her parents brought her to Dr. Allen's clinic only weighing 75 pounds. Allen's first step with his patients was to start them on a fast to completely eliminate the sugar from their body. The fasts usually lasted for several days, depending on the patient, during which time, the patient's urine was checked for sugar. When the amount of sugar in a patient's urine was reduced to an acceptable level, Dr. Allen would gradually reintroduce food, between 400 and 600 calories a day. Under his care, Elizabeth's weight dropped to 55 pounds. She existed on a diet of eggs, lean meat, lettuce, milk, some fruit, and vegetables that were boiled three times to reduce the carbohydrates. Elizabeth was said to have maintained good spirits and followed Dr. Allen's strict lifestyle without complaint. She was discovered "cheating" on her diet only once when she was found in the kitchen after a Thanksgiving dinner, sneaking a piece of turkey skin. I can see Elizabeth standing in the dark kitchen, opening the door of the ice box and with a glance behind her, reaching and pulling a piece of the skin off the turkey that had been cooking all day, filling the house with a smell she could no longer resist.

Dr. Allen kept a strict watch over his patients while they were under his care in the clinic, formulating a specific diet plan for each individual. Many of his patients were not as committed as Elizabeth and were found, "breaking their diet," "sneaking," or "pilfering forbidden foods."

In 1922, Dr. Allen left for Toronto to secure some of the newly discovered insulin. While he was gone, rumors spread among the patients that something momentous was about to happen. One of the nurses, Margate Kienast, describes their reaction:

> . . . *the mere illusion of new hope cajoled patient after patient into new life. Diabetics who had not been out of bed for weeks began to trail weekly about, clinging to walls and furniture. Big stomachs, skin-and-bone necks, skull-like faces, feeble movements, all ages and sexes— they looked like an old Flemish painter's depiction of a resurrection after famine. It was a resurrection, a crawling stirring, as of some vague springtime.*[1]

She remembered the scene when the patients heard that Dr. Allen had come back:

> *We all heard his step coming along the covered walk, past the entrance, to the main hallways. His wife was with him, her quick tapping pace making a queer rhythm with his. The patient's silence concentrated on that sound. When he appeared through the open doorway, he caught the full beseeching of a hundred pairs of eyes. It stopped him dead. Even now, I am sure it was minutes before he spoke to them, his voice curiously mingling concern for his patients with an excitement that he tried his best not to betray.*
>
> *"I think," he said, "I think we have something for you."*[1]

By the time I was diagnosed in the fall of 1985, insulin had been around for decades. I was not going to have to starve myself to stay alive. I would eat, sleep, exercise, and lead an almost normal life. Food was no longer poison, and my diet would not be one of *starvation*. However, the language of the past had influenced the present. Death by starvation was at the root of my disease and so eating was a reward and a punishment; a measure of how far my disease had come. Eating was not about satisfying hunger.

EATING AS A RITUAL/FOOD AND IDENTITY

In the journal *Diabetes Spectrum*, July 2003, "Diabetes and Women's Health Issues," Owens writes:

> *Perceptions of food and cultural meanings attached to food are also concerns that should be addressed, especially for adult women with type 2 diabetes. Maintaining control of diabetes requires making healthy choices when preparing and consuming foods and carrying out other lifestyle changes. However, prescribing lifestyle change for patients with diabetes is challenging and complex because such change requires people to process the historical meaning of food in their culture and its traditions across generations.*

> *For African-American women with type 2 diabetes, for example, modifying their diet may be difficult given the deeply rooted experiences and traditions surrounding food in the African-American culture. Deviating from the traditional food experiences in one's family may be perceived negatively by family members and can result in conflict for people with diabetes.*[2]

THE DIABETES DIET

The language of eating and diabetes has various terms and is constantly changing. Words like "food exchanges" have now been replaced with "carb counting." Low-carb diets can also be called, "low glycemic eating." The words that make up this language are confusing and can feel overwhelming and many women will struggle to find the best cookbook or the right tools to help her manage the food that she eats. In these collected stories you'll see that women use various tools, from carb counting books to websites, to eating the same thing every day to keep their blood sugars from jumping and spiking. There is no perfect solution, and there is a wide range of opinions. Do what works for you.

Eating When Low

Rachel Garlinghouse used to binge when she was low, eating everything but the kitchen sink:

> But of course, that led to a roller coaster of highs and lows for days following. Now, I know to treat a low with a carefully measured amount of juice or three glucose tablets.
>
> I have had many lows in public and usually I sit somewhere, treat my low, and wait for my blood sugar to come up. My most dangerous low occurred when I was in a furniture store. My sugar was 21. I was so out of it that I didn't even feel bad like I normally do with a low. I consumed about eight glucose tablets to bring up my sugar.
>
> Lows are the worst part of my diabetes, and they often occur when a person is trying to maintain tight blood sugar control. Honestly, I would rather my blood sugar run slightly high than slightly low, even though lower blood sugars result in lower A1c numbers. When I am low, I want to eat anything I can get my hands on. Overeating when I'm low feels good at the time; however, the consequences usually entail me waking up high, not being able to work out, and then being high all day. I do get angry with myself when I don't do the right thing, but I have to remember that everyone makes mistakes, and I'm doing a good job managing my disease. When I mess up, I don't wallow in guilt, but instead, get right back into the game.

Lesley Hoffman Goldenberg says she is always hungry:

I am particularly hungry when my sugar is low, or if it was really high and I'm coming down from being high. It hits me, and I get starving from the sudden (or gradual) drop in blood sugar. When that happens, I usually try to eat things like egg whites or nuts so it doesn't affect my sugar dropping.

One of my biggest diabetes pet peeves is when I eat a huge and delicious meal and I'm super full, and then my blood sugar is low. I get so angry! But I clearly have to suck it up and treat with glucose tablets. It just annoys me that I have to consume more calories and I'm already so full. And, yes, I feel incredibly guilty if I over-treat, and I get annoyed when my sugar spikes up later. And yes, I have definitely bolused for a low blood sugar because I've over-treated. That's reality.

Rebecca Walker Bryant almost always over-treats when she is low:

I don't get a "low" feeling now until my blood glucose levels are in the 40s or 50s. I get famished. With my brain spinning and my hands shaking, I will load up on cereal, yogurt, and sweets.

I can recall several times when I have gone out to dinner and then have come home and made a peanut butter and Nutella sandwich on whole wheat bread. It makes me feel horrible. I hate the fact that I can't feel satisfied by my meals. I can't stay away from the pantry. It makes me feel like I am out of control.

Annie Berger used to overeat when she was low because she felt desperate to get her blood sugar up:

It was like my body was screaming at me to keep eating. Afterwards, I felt guilty because I knew I would inevitably end up high later on, and I knew that I wasn't helping my weight at all. While I am always disappointed in myself, I know that the diabetes has that affect on me, and that I probably wouldn't have eaten that way if it weren't for the diabetes.

Learning to Count Carbs

Lesley Hoffman Goldenberg says:

> *When I was first diagnosed, they were still using the exchange system so I think that one exchange was 15 grams of carbs. Eventually, I met with a nutritionist and diabetes educator and learned how to roughly count carbs. It's still a challenge for me, but I'm getting better everyday. I have a few guidebooks that I check once in awhile, and I rely heavily on calorieking.com both for carbohydrate information and calorie information.*

Kristin Makszin started carb counting immediately after her diagnosis:

> *I took a diabetes education class that was mostly geared towards people with type 2 diabetes (I was the only type 1 in the class). I used the* Calorie King *book extensively. I carried it with me everywhere when I was learning. I still have it on my bookshelf, but I rarely need it anymore. When I look over at that beat-up book, it reminds me what a journey it was learning to carb count.*
>
> *Now that I'm aiming for much tighter blood sugar management, I'm counting carbs carefully and I use a Salter scale for accurate carb counting. I now usually determine my carb counts by weight rather than by volume, which I find to be much more reliable.*

Rebecca Walker Bryant says:

> *When I had gestational diabetes, I took a nutrition class and learned to count carbs. Once I was diagnosed and knew that my daughter's health was an issue, I recall that I took a great deal of care and time with my health and diet. I liked counting carbs. It made sense. I am not as careful now. I have worked briefly with nutritionists in the past few years, and wish I could employ one on a full-time basis.*

Dealing With Advice From Others

Annie Berger struggled with coworkers:

> *Prior to getting pregnant, I was trying very hard to stay*
> *away from anything that would spike my blood sugar.*
> *I also don't particularly like cakes, cookies, and so forth*
> *and often don't want to waste my insulin on them. At*
> *work, my coworkers gave me a very hard time about*
> *not eating cake for various team members' birthdays.*
> *I explained why I wasn't eating it but they would keep*
> *pushing me every time a birthday came up. I finally had*
> *to have a very tough discussion with some of them telling*
> *them I refused to discuss it any more and that if they felt*
> *the need to continue to ask me questions and push we*
> *would need to discuss it with HR. I am not the kind of*
> *person who would involve HR over something like this,*
> *but it had gone on a long time and made me very*
> *uncomfortable.*

Lesley Hoffman Goldenberg says:

> *The one thing that annoys the shit out of me (excuse my*
> *language), is when people look at the sugar content of*
> *something for me and tell me it has too much sugar.*
> *I usually look at them, let out a condescending and*
> *sarcastic laugh and say—"I've never in my life looked*
> *at the sugar content of anything. What does that mean*
> *anyway?" They usually have no clue and we move on . . .*
> *oh, and they never do it again.*

Mindful Eating

Sometimes, it's overwhelming to try and figure out how to achieve goals such as weight loss, blood glucose control, and feeling less anxious about having diabetes. We have to think about diabetes with every bite of food we put into our mouths. "Mindful eating" is a term that can help women with diabetes feel more proactive and less emotional when it comes to food. Mindful eating can also get women away from the destructive cycle of focusing on perfection and/or failing to meet the high expectations that are inherent with diabetes care.

There is no single way to start eating mindfully. However, the Center for Mindful Eating, a nonprofit, nonreligious organization created by a group of mindfulness experts, offers the following four principles of mindful eating:

1. Allow yourself to become aware of the positive and nurturing opportunities that are available through food preparation and consumption by respecting your own inner wisdom.
2. Choose to eat food that is both pleasing to you and nourishing to your body by using all your senses to explore, savor, and taste.
3. Acknowledge your responses to food (likes, neutral, or dislikes) without judgment.
4. Learn to be aware of physical hunger and fullness cues to guide your decision when to begin eating and to stop eating.[3]

These principles and more information about the center are available online at http://www.tcme.org.

An important factor of mindful eating is changing the way we think about food. Many women with diabetes have emotionally complex relationships with food and being mindful about eating can help us focus on nourishment and being kind to our bodies.

Michelle Sorensen has food intolerances and says that they have forced her to become more creative in the kitchen:

> *I feel like I enjoy food more than ever. Sometimes,*
> *I indulge in something too sweet but I usually feel tired*
> *and it makes my digestion sluggish . . . . So I get back*
> *on track, because I like feeling healthy.*
>
> *I do, sometimes, meet young women in this situation*
> *as I work as a psychologist and get referrals from the*
> *diabetes community. I encourage them to focus on*
> *evolution of their diet versus revolution (trying to change*
> *everything overnight). I think we need to have compassion*
> *for ourselves when we falter or make mistakes, because*
> *negative self-talk and self-loathing leads to shame, guilt,*
> *anger, and depression . . . those emotions then lead into*

unhealthy coping strategies like overeating or purging. So it all starts with finding love and attending to self-care.

Some women are just far too busy to believe they can cook healthy food versus eating out, and therefore, aren't mindful of what they are feeding themselves. So, whether someone is just having a hard time eating healthy food, or whether they actually struggle with disordered eating, I think women with diabetes have to really examine their lives and schedules and ask themselves if they are prioritizing their health. I withdrew from a PhD program a month before it was about to start. After a year with diabetes, I realized there was no way I could attend to my health and well-being while I met the requirements of that program. I thought I might blame my diabetes and be resentful of that lost opportunity, but now I know I could never regret a decision based on my health. What would be the point of having my doctorate if I wasn't happy? And how can I be happy if I am not healthy? In the long run, even those without a diagnosed health problem are usually happier if they are not overworked and overtired. Diabetes puts an extra onus on self-care and we have to work towards accepting that . . . attending to one's health usually means better energy and vitality, which helps productivity in the long run anyway.

Meal Planning

Imagine a rope that spans from one side of a cliff to the other. (I like to think of the 1980s movie, *Romancing the Stone*, with Michael Douglas and Kathleen Turner.) On one side of the cliff the American Diabetes Association's (ADA) recommendations for diet and meal planning, and the other is Dr. Richard Bernstein's. Each side has its own value. Holding onto this rope as our legs dangle in the air are the people living with diabetes. Some of us are closer to the ADA side and others are closer to Dr. Bernstein's. (There are times in our life when one lifestyle may fit better . . . for example, when a woman is trying to get pregnant or during those certain times of the month when many of us are more insulin resistant, she may find success with Bernstein's low carb methods and other women may prefer to follow the ADA guidelines when it comes to traveling out of the country.) There is a huge variety of styles when it comes to meal planning just as there are a huge variety of women living with diabetes, and there is no one style that fits all.

American Diabetes Association

The ADA recommends the "create your plate" method, which focuses on portion sizes and involves dividing your plate into three sections. The largest section should be filled with "non-starchy vegetables," the next smaller section should be "starchy foods" (such as whole-grain breads, brown rice, beans, etc.), and finally, the smallest section should include protein. "Create your plate" also includes a glass of low-fat milk and a serving of fruit.

The ADA also recommends, carb counting for managing your blood glucose levels:

> *A place to start is at about 45–60 grams of carbohydrate at a meal. You may need more or less carbohydrate at meals depending on how you manage your diabetes. You and your health care team can figure out the right amount for you. Once you know how much carb to eat at a meal, choose your food and the portion size to match.*
>
> *Carbohydrate counting is easier when food labels are available. You can look at how much carbohydrate is in the foods you want to eat and decide how much of the food you can eat. The two most important lines with carbohydrate counting are the serving size and the total carbohydrate amount.*[4]

Dr. Bernstein

Dr. Bernstein was diagnosed in the 1950s with type 1 diabetes when he was 12 years old. Over the years, he has pioneered the controversial ultra low-carb method of management. Dr. Bernstein's philosophy is to keep blood sugars as close to normal as possible with small doses of insulin and very limited use of carbohydrates.

In his book, Dr. Bernstein wrote:

> *If you're going to control your diabetes and get on with a normal life, you will have to change your diet, and the*

when is now. No matter how mild or severe your diabetes, the key aspect of all treatment plans for normalizing blood sugars and preventing or reversing complications of diabetes is diet. In the terms of the Laws of Small Numbers, the single largest "input" you can control is what you eat.

First, eliminate all foods that contain simple sugars. As you should know by now—but it bears repeating—"simple sugar" does not mean just table sugar; that's why, I prefer to call them fast-acting carbohydrates. Most breads and other starchy foods, such as potatoes and grains, become glucose so rapidly that they can cause serious postprandial increases in blood sugar.

Second, limit your total carbohydrate intake to an amount that will work with your injected insulin or your body's remaining phase II insulin response, if any. In this way, you avoid a postprandial blood sugar increase, and avoid overworking any remaining insulin-producing beta cells of your pancreas (research has demonstrated that beta cell burnout can be slowed or halted by normalizing blood sugars).

Third, stop eating when you no longer feel hungry, not when you're stuffed. There's no reason for you to leave the table hungry, but there's also no reason to be gluttonous.[5]

Dr. Bernstein's books, *The Diabetes Diet* and *The Diabetes Solution*, include information about his dietary guidelines. Although his approach is definitely not for everyone, he is a living proof that his meal planning works, and he also acknowledges its challenges:

Most of my patients initially feel somewhat deprived, but also grateful because they feel more alert and healthier. I fall into this category myself. My mouth waters whenever I pass a bakery shop and sniff the aroma of fresh bread, but I am also grateful simply to be alive and sniffing.[5]

Natural Eating

Michelle Sorensen was diagnosed with type 1 diabetes 11 years ago, a few weeks before her 25th birthday:

> *I was in the middle of graduate school and had felt unwell the entire school year. For a week before I was diagnosed, I was so dehydrated that I could barely speak without drinking. I was exhausted and desperately thirsty. I finally took myself to the Toronto General Hospital (the place where Banting and Best first injected patients with insulin). There, I received my type 1 diabetes diagnosis and my first insulin in an IV drip. And thus, began the long process of adapting to my diabetes.*

> *Initially, I focused on being "the perfect diabetic." After about 6 months of carbohydrate counting, writing down all of my blood sugar levels, and battling the physical symptoms of hypoglycemia and hyperglycemia, I felt decades older than my peers. And as I approached the 1-year anniversary of my diagnosis and relived the trauma of the year before, I felt depressed and overwhelmed.*

> *From the time I was diagnosed, I'd also suffered from gastrointestinal symptoms. But I did not have the energy to focus on anything other than my diabetes management and finishing my degree in psychology. I was then accepted into a PhD program, but a month before school started, I withdrew. I felt I could not take care of my health and continue with my studies.*

> *Traditional medical approaches and referrals did not help me to understand my digestive problems. After a few more years of living with uncomfortable gastrointestinal issues, and then a period of worsening symptoms, I decided it was time to give naturopathy a chance.*

> *My naturopathologist quickly identified a number of food intolerances causing my digestive upset, mood instability, and symptoms of fatigue. When I went through my list and saw [that] I needed to eliminate wheat, gluten, dairy, eggs*

and some of my favorite vegetables and fruit, I wondered what I would eat. But after so many years of feeling ill, I was willing to do anything to feel better.

My first step was to eliminate the allergens. The worst of my GI symptoms resolved over the course of the first 6–12 months on my new diet. I no longer experienced acute pain, and the constant heartburn I had suffered from started to subside. Overall, I felt about 80 percent better. I ate more and more vegan food during my first pregnancy. I developed an addiction to green juice and relished my huge salads, along with dehydrated buckwheat pizzas, "pasta" made from vegetable spirals, and amazing desserts. I took an active approach to improving my health. I consulted with a raw food specialist for tips on incorporating more nutrition into my diet. My husband and I decided to start our day with a green smoothie for two weeks and see how we felt. When I started drinking the green smoothies, I noticed how much more stable my sugars were throughout the mornings. Having a carbohydrate-based breakfast had always led to highs in the morning. Another important change was that I craved greens, vegetables, and healthy food all day long. I became pregnant again, and had a lot of motivation to eat well.

My sugar control has vastly improved on a vegan, plant-based diet. I believe a lot of my difficulty with glucose control overnight stemmed from the unpredictability of meat that was digested hours after being eaten, leading to a spike in my sugars while I slept. Eating fewer refined, starchy foods has been crucial to better control too. I need less insulin with meals, meaning that I am not chasing high sugars and then crashing low all the time. And without those highs and lows, I feel healthier and happier.

Over the last 7 years, I have changed my lifestyle and focused my energy on what makes me and my family happy. It is not my fault that I developed diabetes, but my health is my responsibility, and so I do everything I can to create a happy, healthy life.

QUESTIONS AND ANSWERS WITH
ELIZABETH STEPHENS AND LYNDSAY RIFFE

What are your thoughts on low-carb eating?

Dr. Stephens says: Well, in a totally unscientific way, I think low-carb eating is often really helpful for glucose control. Large, high-carb meals are often really tough to effectively bolus for (even if you know exactly how much carb is in it, the absorption can be unpredictable), so trying to eat fewer carbs is helpful, especially for postprandial blood glucose. But the limitation, of course, is what you add as the other nutrient; [that is], high fat foods, which can add calories and, in the long haul, have a poor effect on lipids. Protein often travels with fat, and you have to be careful if you have renal issues—so I don't have a great answer for all situations, but I would say I try to recommend "lower" carb diets than [what] the ADA and many dietitians suggest.

Lyndsay Riffe says: I recommend my patients to do their best [in] eating consistent carbohydrates, and avoid overloading the body with too many carbohydrates at one time. At the same time, I recommend the American Diabetes Association and American Dietetics Association's stance to consume approximately 40–50 percent of calories from carbohydrates, while stressing the *choice* of carbohydrates people consume. The minimal carbohydrate amount to fuel the brain and body is 130 grams of carbs per day. Restrictive diets (low-carb diets) are typically non-sustainable. My experience talking with those that have followed a low-carb diet is they cannot maintain it, and end up gaining all the weight back and then some. Furthermore, low-carb diets do not coincide with a heart-healthy diet, which is important for the person with diabetes.

Women with diabetes have an increased risk of developing celiac disease, do you counsel anyone with celiac disease and if so, what are your recommendations?

Lyndsay Riffe says: Research has shown [that] celiac disease and type 1 diabetes share similar genes. Approximately 1 percent of the general population has celiac disease, where 2 percent of those with type 1 diabetes also have celiac disease, and 10 percent of pediatric diabetes population have both type 1 and celiac. Some diabetes clinics do routine screening for celiac disease, due to the connection between the two autoimmune diseases. At the same time, many go undiagnosed with celiac disease, as symptoms may not be as obvious. Personally, I do agree people with diabetes should routinely be screened for celiac disease. The diet restricts all gluten products, which includes wheat, barley, and rye, while oats are controversial. Persons are encouraged to follow the diet strictly, to avoid damage to villi, which can cause long-term problems like anemia, osteoporosis, [and so forth]. Patients should be encouraged to consume fruits, vegetables, beans, lean meats, and healthy fats. The market for gluten-free products is continuing to grow, which helps those with celiac disease have more options. However, a lot of those products can be non-healthy choices such as other refined carbohydrate options.

Do you use the glycemic index with your patients? If so, can you explain the benefits?

Lyndsay Riffe says: The glycemic index is a measure of how quickly an individual food is digested into glucose. Looking at the glycemic index alone is not useful, as the quantity of the food consumed, as well as what that food is consumed with, can affect the glycemic response. Furthermore, glycemic response of foods can vary from one person to the next. I encourage patients to develop their own "list" of glycemic response. There are many factors that affect the glycemic response, such as fat, protein, fiber, cooking, and how much the food has been processed. Generally speaking, foods containing fiber and minimally processed foods have a lower glycemic response and are part of a healthy diet. Healthy fats such as avocado, olive oil, and nuts, as well as lean protein choices, can help balance out the effect of a meal's glycemic response.

What do you think about vegan/natural eating for people with diabetes?

Lyndsay Riffe says: In general, eating more of a plant-based diet assists with weight management, blood sugar management, and cardiovascular health.

I know that, as diabetics, we lose the ability to regulate hunger, because we don't produce amylin. Therefore, in order to replicate the body's natural response to eating and becoming full, many doctors prescribe Symlin. What are your thoughts/recommendations on this topic?

Lyndsay Riffe says: Amylin is a hormone that partners with insulin, so those who are making little or no insulin are also not making amylin. Symlin is the medication option for those that want to replace amylin. Symlin tells your brain that you are fuller at meals, while also slows down how quickly your food digests and reduces how much glucose your liver makes. Symlin is beneficial for reducing post-meal spikes in blood sugar, because not only does that individual get glucose from the carbohydrate-containing foods consumed, their body also continues to release glucose from the liver (double stacking!). Those that take Symlin typically need less insulin. However, there is not a one size fits all recommendation. People tend to get frustrated with figuring out the right insulin dose when on Symlin, the best advice is to try to not expect perfection after using a few times, it takes time! Although it is supposed to be dosed with all meals, one can take it 1–2 times per day during their more problematic times of the day.

AUTHENTIC ADVICE

■ Rebecca Walker Bryant says:
Take diabetes seriously. Learn all that you can in the beginning. There are people out there who want and can help you. It does help to write it down. I [write in my] journal every day. Also, know what you can and cannot control. My only issue is my high blood sugars. I am lucky to not have to deal with high cholesterol and blood pressure at this point. I am, however, already dealing with complications of high blood sugars: neuropathy in my stomach and legs. Why I already have this, it is not clear. Good control is worth every bit of the long, healthy life you reap from it.

■ Annie Berger says:

Insulin and treatment is so advanced now that there is no reason for you to feel that you need to go on a "diabetes diet" and change your whole life right away. Learn how to make insulin adapt to your life, not how to make your life adapt to the diabetes. Of course, there may be certain things you should avoid or others you should eat more, but don't get overwhelmed in the beginning thinking that everything you eat had to change drastically.

■ Rachel Garlinghouse says:

I volunteer at a hospital and have some interaction with diabetes patients. I also am approached almost daily by someone who is either newly diagnosed or knows someone who is. I advise them to learn to read nutrition labels and ingredients lists. One cannot rely on another person (a medical professional, a clever advertiser, etc.) to constantly tell them the best way to eat. My motto: Knowledge is power. Diabetes is 99 percent managed by the patient.

4 Eating Disorders and Body Image

The dining hall of my boarding school was in the same building as the basketball court, locker rooms, and the athletic department, and the stench of sweat-soaked equipment always mingled with the spaghetti sauce and garlic bread from the kitchen. One night, during the fall of my sophomore year, I stood in the line for dinner behind Kate, a girl from New York City. She turned around and asked if I wanted to study biology with her that night. I was thrilled because she was popular. She was rich, beautiful, and always surrounded by a group of friends. I remember watching her fill her plate with noodles and meat sauce and thought, maybe just this once, taking a ladle full of the "forbidden noodles."

I followed her to her table and then we sat down to eat spaghetti. When she went back for seconds, I was surprised, but followed her again. I had diabetes for only a year, but I knew spaghetti was on the "bad list" of foods at 42 grams of carbs per serving. But it tasted so good that I ate every drop of the thick tomato sauce with warm, spicy meatballs and crunchy garlic bread (24 grams) dripping with butter. I wondered if Kate knew that I was diabetic and not supposed to eat all this food. When we cleaned our plates again, ignoring everyone else at the table, Kate said it was time to go so I followed her out of the dining hall and down the path toward her dorm to study.

When we got to her dorm, she said that she was going to order pizza. I remembered thinking that that was strange, because I was already full from the pasta, but I was thrilled to be hanging out with her and didn't ask any questions. After a while, the pizza arrived (20 grams of carbs per slice; pizza is *high on the glycemic index and can cause unstable blood glucose levels*), and the smell filled the room. I couldn't resist. I wasn't hungry, but I took the slice that Kate handed me. We talked about biology, and when the pizza was gone, Kate said she wanted a dessert. Grabbing my arm, we walked across the campus to the mini-mart. Kate bought Ben & Jerry's ice cream (18 grams of carbs per serving) and cigarettes. I was full and knew the ice cream would be too much, that my blood sugar would sky rocket, but Kate reached over and grabbed my elbow, guiding me up the steps of her dorm. We ate the ice cream side by side on her bed with our biology book open in front of us. When the tub of ice cream was empty, Kate said, "let's go," I didn't ask any questions.

We walked through the dark streets of the campus. The tree-lined road was empty and growing dark. I looked around and wondered where everyone was. Where were the teachers who would ask us what we were doing, and why weren't we in study hall? We reached the art building and I followed Kate to the bathroom. She opened the door and turned on a light. The room was small and on the counter, there were paint brushes left out to dry. With the door closed and locked, I felt claustrophobic, but there was nowhere to go. Kate reached under the cabinet and pulled out a toothbrush. "Will you hold it?" she said. She meant her hair. I must have looked at her strangely because after that she said, "I'm not going to get fat from all that food, are you?" I grabbed a fistful of her thick brown hair while she leaned over the toilet, and then shoved the toothbrush down her throat and gagged. The sound echoed off the walls and the food we'd eaten sat like a cement brick in my stomach. She gagged again and again, flushing each time after she'd thrown up. I closed my eyes. When she was done, I let go of her hair. Kate splashed water on her face and handed me an extra toothbrush.

"Your turn," she said. I realized that her stomach was emptied out, free of all the calories we'd consumed, and that mine would stay full.

My instinct was to say that I couldn't throw up what I'd eaten because I had diabetes, but I knew that diabetes also meant that I should never have eaten all that food in the first place. But it felt so good to eat without thinking, to eat the foods that were on the bad list: pasta, pizza, and ice cream. Foods that I'd missed on my restricted diet, foods that tasted so good. Eating those foods with Kate was my first diabetes rebellion and for a brief time, it felt good. But walking back to my dorm in the dark, my stomach bloated, I realized what I'd done and was scared. I was scared of getting low, scared of being high, and scared that having diabetes meant that I couldn't follow Kate's footsteps.

For years, I wondered why Kate picked me that night. I wondered if she saw something in me and knew that I would follow her, or maybe, she knew that I wouldn't ask any questions. Did she see the way I looked at the food in the dining hall, the way my eyes filled with longing? Had she been watching me?

Eating disorders are nearly twice as common in young women with type 1 diabetes as their healthy peers. A nurse at Duke University says:

> *By the time of diabetes diagnosis or during periods of poor metabolic control, there may be a loss of weight. For some young women in the immediate preteen or early teen years, this weight loss may be perceived to be highly desirable. However, the introduction of insulin treatment or improved metabolic control inevitably leads to weight gain, which may negatively affect the vulnerable teen.*

I'd lost 15 pounds in less than a week on my already thin frame when I was diagnosed, and as I search through my photographs from those years, I try to see a change in my body size. I never became heavy but I began to write in my journal about wanting to be thin. The language in my writing begins to reflect a rapidly diminishing sense of self-worth.

> *Another common theme relates to feeling ashamed or stigmatized about having diabetes. The attention to body, eating, and planning to eat required for good diabetes care may be in opposition to the eating disorder beliefs that bodily needs are shameful and that denying oneself of food is morally laudable.*

What would I have been like if I was never diagnosed? What would my relationship to my body and to food have been like if I'd stayed healthy? I wondered.

Every time I stood in line at the dining hall, I thought about that night with Kate. I watched her walking from her table up to the bathroom and knew what she was going to do. Every time I tested my blood sugar, gave myself a shot, and ate, whether I was hungry or not, I thought about Kate. I pushed the food around on my plate, for I was not hungry, and then, I swallowed some food, not tasting it.

Dr. Ann Goebel-Fabbri, an instructor in psychiatry at Harvard Medical School and an investigator on Behavioral and Mental Health at the

Joslin Diabetes Center, is an expert in the field of diabetes and eating disorders. She says:

> *So much attention to food is required and taught by diabetes educators, they're trying to come up with a more flexible way of teaching this and a less morally judgmental way of teaching this, but it still gets misconstrued, and it's not ever going to be a normal relationship with food because there's all these calculations that have to be done. With old style diabetes management, before the days of "designer insulins," you had to eat at certain times of day, whether you were hungry or not. Patients unlearned their body's usual response to hunger, and had to eat according to requirements.*

As women with diabetes, we must learn to listen to our bodies and develop a heightened awareness with our body's signals. And because our bodies often give us mixed signals (such as when our blood sugar is on the rise and we become very hungry), this relationship is not innate; it is learned through trial and error. Dr. Goebel-Fabbri says that many women experience a feeling of betrayal and may try to control some aspect of their lives that does feel controllable. This aspect is often food.

Rachel Garlinghouse says:

> *I am a control freak in many areas of my life, and I think this has served me well when it comes to my diet. I carefully choose all my foods, good or bad! If I'm going to indulge, I do so by making sure I'm getting exactly what I want. For example, I could care less about a bag of chips but brownies? Bring them on! So I don't eat the chips and the brownies. I'll portion out my dessert (in a one-cup bowl) and enjoy it!*

EATING DISORDER STATISTICS/FACTS

- Researchers estimate that 10–20 percent of girls in their mid-teen years and 30–40 percent of late-teenage girls, and young adult women with diabetes skip or alter insulin doses to control their weight.

- The mortality rate from diabetes alone is roughly 2.5 percent annually. For anorexia nervosa, it is 6.5 percent. But patients with diabulimia—which is referred to, in health care circles, as *dual diagnosis*—have a mortality rate of 34.8 percent per year.
- According to anecdotal research that was done at Park Nicollet, patients with diabulimia routinely suffer from retinopathy, neuropathy, metabolic imbalance, depression and other mood disorders, kidney disease, and heart attacks.
- Self-reported insulin restriction conveyed a threefold increased risk of mortality during 11-year follow up.

Possible Causes/Risk Factors:

- The cycle of inexact insulin dosing can cause weight gain, which increases insulin requirements and resistance. And there's another factor at work: The insulin-producing cells that were attacked by the disease also make amylin, which works with other appetite regulating hormones, such as leptin, to regulate the sensation of fullness. The resulting difficulty of diabetics to determine whether they are full has been documented in anorexia. A behavioral health psychologist who's research specializes in psychosocial aspects of types 1 and 2 diabetes and obesity in children and adolescents says, "Destruction of β-cells results in the inability to secrete both insulin and amylin, contributing to dysregulation of appetite and satiety."
- Interestingly, most type 1 diabetics lose a lot of weight before diagnosis because they excrete rather than metabolize calories. For months, they may be able to eat large amounts of food and not gain any weight. When they start taking insulin to "control" their disease, they can gain a lot of weight quickly.
- Loss of control because of required monitoring and reporting of food intake, physical activity, and blood glucose
- Loss of autonomy because of parental/spousal/familial concern/ vigilance regarding health status
- Increased perfectionism because of the accountability to health care providers regarding self-care behaviors and glycemic status
- Lower self-esteem and body image after diagnosis

■ The CDC report states that the stress related to having a chronic illness can exacerbate other difficulties for both the patient and the family and make the eruption of a latent eating disorder more likely. Persons with diabetes who are struggling with issues of identity or adjustment brought about by the diagnosis of a chronic illness are at higher risk of developing eating disorders than are those who are coping fairly well with life.

Rachel Garlinghouse says:

I lost about 35 pounds during the year and a half I went undiagnosed. I was wearing a size zero (and all those clothes were too big). The initial weight loss yielded a lot of compliments; however, after I started to lose pound after pound, I began to look like a person who had been in a concentration camp. My hair was thinning, my skin was yellow in color, and I had no energy. At my lowest point, I was 96 pounds, which is 42 pounds under the normal weight for a person of my height. I was very depressed, and it only got worse with the nasty comments I heard constantly. One man at my gym walked by me, gave me the up and down look, and said, "Eat a hamburger." People, including my own doctor, believed I had anorexia. I realized how alone a young woman with an eating disorder must feel, and the comments only made the situation worse.

After my diagnosis, I gained about 50 pounds in a year and a half. It was incredibly depressing to go from "normal" (prediabetes), to drastically underweight, to weighing more than I ever had in my life. My weight is now steady at 140 pounds, which is normal for a woman of my height. I do wish I weighed about 10 pounds less sometimes; however, I know that health and my mental stability are far more important than a number on a scale. I exercise daily, I make healthy food choices, and I model healthy behaviors for my family, especially my young daughter.

Michelle Sorensen was a little underweight when she was diagnosed:

I had always been petite but in those months leading up to the diagnosis, I ate and drank so much, but was quite thin. My biggest weight loss came at the time of the 1-year anniversary of my diagnosis. I had become quite depressed, was not eating enough, and was stressed about a relationship I was in at the time. Plus, I was diagnosed in the middle of my masters, so I was about to start my PhD, and was struggling to finish my master's thesis, and got thinner and thinner. I have always had pretty stable weight and a healthy approach to managing weight, but I knew I was getting obsessive about the number on the scale. I literally felt like it was the one thing I could control. As I got thinner, I felt an odd sense of satisfaction . . . I would look at my stomach, with bruises from injections, and I could see the bones in my back and hips . . . and I remember thinking, "Yes, now I look sick." Diabetes is a strange disease, because you can be in crisis with your health and you look so normal. It is a blessing on the one hand, but if you aren't good at asking for help, it also means everyone will think you are fine when you are not. Luckily, I got past that stage and started to gain weight back. I went on the pump about 2 years after my diagnosis and initially gained some weight from that change because I had such newfound freedom in when I ate and how much. I overcompensated a bit for the years of restriction!

SIGNS AND SYMPTOMS OF DISORDERED EATING

- Women repeatedly not bringing their meter into doctor appointments
- Unexplained weight changes
- Gradually increased A1c
- Recurrent yeast infections
- Recurrent diabetic ketoacidosis (DKA)

EATING DISORDER DIAGNOSES

One behavioral psychologist believes, "You can't use the same criteria to diagnose eating disorders that you use in nondiabetic populations because what we actually prescribe as part of diabetes treatment is part of disordered eating behavior."

Types of Eating Disorders

Dr. Ann Goebel-Fabbri says:

> *In general, there are higher rates of bulimia across the board. What I tend to see are people who are somewhere in between and that's true for all eating disorders. The largest diagnostic group of eating disorder groups is called "eating disorder not otherwise specified" (EDNOS), and it describes the way various symptoms of eating disorders can ebb and flow. What I see most is women desiring a very thin body, and coming at that desire through a variety of dangerous means.*

Diabulimia

Diabulimia is characterized by a person with diabetes who is intentionally skipping insulin therapy to keep blood glucose levels elevated, which in turn causes dangerous weight loss. Dr. Goebel-Fabbri doesn't like this term because she says it is offensive and forces these complicated illnesses into one term.

Symptoms of diabulimia include:

- Excessive exercise
- Intentionally skipped or drastically lowered insulin doses
- Decreased blood glucose monitoring
- Rapid weight loss
- Excessive urination
- Vomiting
- Extreme concern with body weight and shape

Anorexia Nervosa

Anorexia nervosa is characterized by self-starvation and excessive weight loss, and the following symptoms:

- Refusal to maintain body weight at or above the minimum normal weight based on height, body type, age, and activity level

- Intense fear of weight gain or being fat
- Feeling fat or overweight despite dramatic weight loss
- Loss of menstrual periods
- Extreme concern with body weight and shape
- Disturbance of perception and fixation on a specific body part

Bulimia Nervosa

Bulimia nervosa is characterized by a secretive cycle of binge eating followed by purging. Bulimia includes eating large amounts of food—more than most people would eat in one meal—in short periods, then getting rid of the food and calories through vomiting, laxative abuse, or overexercising.

- Repeated episodes of binging and purging
- Feeling out of control during a binge and eating beyond the point of comfortable fullness
- Purging after a binge (typically by self-induced vomiting, abuse of laxatives, diet pills and/or diuretics, excessive exercise, or fasting)
- Frequent dieting
- Extreme concern with body weight and shape
- Sense of loss of control in eating

The CDC report states that the central issue for persons with bulimia nervosa is a feeling of living behind a facade. An adolescent girl with bulimia tends to believe that everyone thinks she is pretty, mature, and capable. She fears that others will find out that she is not really that perfect and will be angry and disappointed with herself. Although perfect blood glucose control is not a realistic expectation for persons with diabetes, adolescent girls with bulimia and diabetes need to present a facade of perfection to hide their failure from parents and health care providers. Thus, bulimic girls with diabetes frequently report excellent blood glucose control and "no difficulties" with diabetes management but have very elevated hemoglobin A1c levels.

MYTHS AND STEREOTYPES

- Insulin makes you fat.
- You're cheating (when you eat something "unacceptable").

■ You can't eat that, you have diabetes.

■ You got diabetes because you ate too much sugar.

Risks

"I think of risks in two ways," Dr. Goebel-Fabbri says. "One is the immediate risks which include DKA [and] infections, but also longer term complications of diabetes happening more frequently in younger ages."

■ Extremely high A1c test results
■ Frequent bouts of and hospitalizations for poor blood sugar control
■ Anxiety about or avoidance of being weighed
■ Frequent requests to switch meal-planning approaches
■ Frequent severe low blood sugar
■ Widely fluctuating blood sugar levels without obvious reasons
■ Delay in puberty, sexual maturation, or irregular or no menses
■ Binging with food or alcohol at least twice a week for 3 months
■ Exercise more than what is necessary to stay fit
■ Severe family stress

Ann Rosenquist Fee learned to "starve down" her blood sugars:

Sixteen years into my diagnosis, at age 41, I'm not quite ready to let go of the games I play with food in order to outsmart my A1c. If we were talking about anything else, any other aspect of living with diabetes, I could sit down with a newly diagnosed friend or stranger and offer support and compassion and funny little anecdotes that would surely put her at ease. With any other piece, I'd be the first to help her feel that we're in this together, and my triumphs and mistakes are open to her as she finds her way.

Not with eating. Those games are private, because I still play from time to time. They're not yet anecdotes. They're just confessions.

For more than a decade, I kept my A1cs within the nondiabetic range by "starving down" my sugars. I learned that term from the general practitioner who first told me to stop doing it and to gain 5 pounds so my periods would start again after a year of amenorrhea. (I did, and they did.) My standard practice was to overdose just slightly on short-acting insulin, then chase the lows with glucose tablets. And then chase any subsequent highs with an extra shot, or 20 minutes with a Hula-Hoop.

At first, I could feel lows in the 70s, but over time, I quit sweating, shaking, or feeling it at all until about 50. That meant a lot of testing to know when it was time for a tablet. I also ate the same things every day at the same times as much as possible, mostly protein, sometimes just plain yogurt, and cottage cheese all day for all 6 tiny meals. Sometimes I added sunflower seeds and Equal. I tried to eat where my husband and my son couldn't see, because I knew it looked silly, if not crazy. I also knew I was thin but that wasn't the point. The point was not going blind or ending up on dialysis due to too many high postprandials, too many carbs. When I saw high numbers on my meter, I choked up. I didn't even know what dialysis involved, but I pictured myself hooked up to some machine in a crappy storefront in a strip mall, with a sign like "Southern Minnesota Dialysis" out in front. I imagined the room would smell of urine and that it would be a beautiful fall day outside while I lay trapped, remembering the normal meals that sent me there. So the choice seemed clear, and I made it, one glucose chaser at a time.

That didn't mix well with social life. I remember one meal in particular with my husband and some friends at a Denny's or Perkins or some place like that. I ordered pancakes like a regular person, and I didn't know how much insulin to take or that a postprandial over 120 was probably fine just this once. We hung around in the booth a long time after the meal, which meant my insulin sat there pooling under my belly skin, not doing its job at all. I tested about an hour after we ate and was above 200, and I got mad and took some Novolog and went outside to walk around the parking lot. My husband was great and so were our friends but my self-flagellation kind of killed the party.

It felt better to me to see a 72 or 54 an hour after eating and treat it fast with a tablet or two, than to worry about long-term damage. Lows made me sweaty and blurry for a few minutes, but that seemed preferable to inviting neuropathy or blindness. With lows, I was just uncomfortable. I wasn't doing any real harm. And my A1cs stayed in that lovely perfect range.

This past year, I mentioned to my new endocrinologist that I'd been having trouble remembering details—names, meeting times, feeling sure I'd just sent the right email to the right colleague, things like that. I told her it felt physical, like details just didn't stick anymore despite that I'd always been a detail person. I wasn't menopausal or particularly stressed or anything like that. Just newly batty, kind of a constant low-grade blur. I asked her if all that hypoglycemia for that decade or so could have had anything to do with it. She said she knew of new research suggesting that frequent lows lead to short-term memory loss. I could try ginkgo biloba to maintain my brain, but there was really nothing to do at this point except avoid further damage by avoiding lows.

I'm not saying my food games worked. They were a bad idea the same way too much whiskey is a bad idea. But even now, despite the cost, I can't dismiss the hope and power those games gave me—and sometimes still give me—in the moment. It feels good to see an 83, better than it feels to see a 175, and the short-term relief still makes it easy sometimes to turn down a lunch date and stay home with a bowl of cottage cheese and a Hula-Hoop. It would be cruel and unhealthy to advise those kinds of games. But if a newly diagnosed friend or stranger confessed to starving down her sugars because it felt like her only foothold in the very private climb up and out of a dead-pancreas-shaped pit, I'd tell her she wasn't alone.

DEPRESSION AND EATING DISORDERS

Lee Ann Thill was 5 years old when she was diagnosed. She hadn't been feeling well and her mom promised her a trip to Kentucky Fried Chicken. Instead, they ended up at the hospital. As an only child of a single mother, Lee Ann says that she was on her own a great deal. She remembers sneaking a jellybean after being told that she couldn't eat any sugar, and when she ate it, she was afraid she was going to die:

> *My dad's side of the family lived in Texas and ate traditional southern foods. I was the kid who would eat anything, and my family loved that about me. I spent summers with my dad in Texas and was living in this environment where everyone wanted me to eat, so this kind of set the stage for my eating disorder. My mom was initially really "neurotic" about my food until the doctors told her to relax. She would let me have treats on occasion, like cake on birthdays. She didn't keep stuff from me, but there was definitely a forbidden sense to food. In the 1st grade, I remember that I had to have a snack in my classroom. I sat at the table by myself while the other kids went out for recess. After a while, I started skipping the snacks and hiding them in my desk. One morning, I ended up having a seizure in class, and the teacher found the food I'd hidden and I got into trouble.*

> *When I was 12 my mom and I moved to Pennsylvania, and I laid down the law with her, I said nobody is going to know about my diabetes. I wanted a fresh start. I didn't want to go through the isolation I experienced in grade school. I was always subconsciously gauging people to see who I could trust to tell them about my diabetes. My concern was that they [were] going to tell other people, I had a fear of being singled out and being different, diabetes was fodder for teasing.*

> *In the summer I returned to Texas and went to diabetes camp where I flourished. I was a different person at camp; it was so freeing to not be looking over my shoulder all the time. At home, I wasn't popular but at camp, I was like the head cheerleader. Depression runs in my family and looking*

back, I can see that it was starting to take hold of me even before my diagnosis. No one noticed how bad I was struggling, and if they did, maybe they didn't know what to do. The attitude at home was to carry on and deal with the crap in your life. My mom did understand the importance of camp and made sure I could return summer after summer.

I gained a lot of weight during the summer of 8th grade. When I returned home from camp, my mom said, "What happened to you? You have to lose weight." I began to exercise 3 to 4 times a day and became obsessed with dieting. I felt like I was rejected by my friends because of the weight gain. That Halloween, I went trick or treating with a friend and ate a lot of candy, and it was the first time I tried to make myself throw up. I remember reading Seventeen *magazine about girls with bulimia, and then, there were the girls at diabetes camp who were skipping shots, so I learned about insulin restriction and binging. I associated insulin with weight gain.*

By the next summer, Lee Ann didn't go to camp, and her depression worsened. She was eating, throwing up, skipping shots, and sleeping. "It was an effort for me to do anything," she says. Her mom was not seeing the reality of what was happening, and in a call for help, Lee Ann induced DKA so that she could go to the hospital. In the hospital for a couple of days, she missed school and it was a vicious cycle. She got more behind and figured, "I can't even catch up." She attempted suicide and ended up in the ER and ICU. Lee Ann was 16 years old at the time and spent Christmas at the psychiatric unit of the hospital. She continued to struggle with eating disorders and depression and went on meds, but "eating disorders took a good prominent hold on me," she said.

Eventually, Lee Ann went to graduate school, and met her husband who inspired her to change her life. She still had a fear of taking insulin and gaining weight but began seeing an endocrinologist, because she was scared that her choices were catching up with her. Her A1cs were in the 8–9 percent and she couldn't stop throwing up, but for the first time, she wanted to change:

At 32 years old, I went into treatment again and was asked for the first time, how my diabetes affected my

*emotions. When I began talking about diabetes, I saw
how I related to others and how it affected my life.
I addressed a lot of those issues in therapy and finally
stopped throwing up. There were a lot of lost opportunities along the way that failed to address what was at the
heart of my depression and eating disorder. I had been
in denial for years and was not connecting the feelings I
had about diabetes with the way I was physically beating
myself up.*

Living a Double Life

Charla was chubby as a kid and remembers being picked on and hating
it. As someone who was always aware of how much she was eating,
when she was 16 years old and began losing weight and eating all she
wanted, she was thrilled:

*God was answering my prayers! I also couldn't get out of
bed and knew something was wrong. My parents eventually took me to the hospital and I was diagnosed with type
1 diabetes in 1974. In the hospital for a week, I gained
14 pounds. I felt like the Michelin man. I was given a list of
food exchanges and told what I could and couldn't eat and
sent home. I remember thinking, I can't do this. The day
I got out of the hospital, I started skipping insulin because
I had to lose the weight.*

*In high school, I didn't want to be different from my
friends. I felt different because of my family (growing up
in an alcoholic family) and my illness. So I kept diabetes a
secret—which turned into a life-long pattern. I had a
double life. I worked very hard to keep my diabetes a
secret. Being open was very hard for me. I didn't want
anyone to know for multiple reasons. I was ashamed and
felt different. I was afraid boys wouldn't want to date me
and marry me (remember I was 16) because I was either
going to die or be sick with all kinds of things. Other
people wouldn't want to be friends because of all my
restrictions, that I wouldn't be any fun if I followed my*

diet. And I also felt stupid and bad for not following my diet. (What was wrong with me?)

By the time I was in college, I started throwing up my food. I thought, if I don't swallow the food, then it won't raise my blood sugars . . . I continued skipping shots and ended up in DKA more than once. The first time I was in the hospital, they told me, "Don't skip your insulin or you'll die," and that scared the living daylights out of me. So I decided that I would take enough insulin to survive because taking insulin meant gaining weight. I would take one shot at bedtime because asleep, I didn't have to think about the insulin causing me to gain weight. My college roommates used to monitor my food and tell me I couldn't eat certain items, so I would "sneak" and "cheat."

I remember being given all kinds of scary books when I was diagnosed, about how I was going to die by the time I was 30, so I thought, "why worry?" I'm going to live fast and die young. I'm going to eat what I want to and do what I want to and I'm going to die enjoying my life. I stopped throwing up but was still omitting insulin because it was so much nicer (than throwing up). I thought, if I don't pay attention to it, then I don't have diabetes.

I wanted to be skinny so I could go to the beach or go play tennis, but I couldn't get myself up off the couch to go play tennis. I know now that I didn't have the coping skills to deal with the stressors of my life, so I ate.

I thought that I had to be perfect; I had to have blood sugars of 120 mg/dl and if I couldn't make that happen, why bother? I didn't test because I knew it was going to be high. I was the worst diabetic in the world.

In her 30s, Charla began having complications in her eyes—diabetic retinopathy. She avoided doctors like the plague because they yelled at her:

I can remember thinking to myself, Charla, what is it going to take before you quit this self-destructive behavior?

*Going blind was not enough to stop me; I couldn't quit.
I didn't quit. I continued looking for help; however, thinking there's got to be some way I can learn to accept this
disease, I can't give up. But I was alone, with no family
support, no support from my doctors (I was labeled
"noncompliant"). I hated it. I hated anything to do with
diabetes; any time I thought about diabetes, it made me
sad. I went to ADA conferences and felt frustrated, because
everyone there seemed to be the perfect diabetics, which
made me feel more alone and more like a bad diabetic.
Nobody was complaining that they had diabetes or that
they didn't like it. I tried overeaters support groups,
therapy and eating disorder support groups but they all
told me, "Don't think about food, only eat when you're
hungry." When you have diabetes you think about food
all the time!*

Finally, Charla found a female endocrinologist who worked with her
to get her on a healthy track. Finding a supportive doctor made a big difference. Charla also discovered the Behavioral Diabetes Institute in San
Diego. She was taught cognitive behavioral therapy (CBT) coping skills
and began making progress but "still couldn't get the diabetes thing
down." Charla also went on a pump, which was difficult at first, but
made a big difference in the end:

*When I first started wearing the pump, I hated it. I felt
like it was a scarlet D on my head. I almost gave it back.
I stopped wearing dresses. I hated wearing it on my belt
because you could see the tubing, so I started wearing
baggy blouses that I could pull up, so the blouse would
hang over and cover it, and baggier pants. Cruel dilemma,
I wanted to be thin, but I had to wear clothes that made
me look bigger. Then I figured out I could hide it in a
pants pocket by putting a hole in the pocket and stringing
the tubing through the hole. Once I figured that out, it was
much better, but then it still came up when I would meet
someone new. I'm glad I stuck with it.*

*I'm still a stubborn person and I still fight, but now it's
fighting to take care of myself to win against diabetes.*

All the energy I used to put into hating my diabetes, now I use to take care of myself. My life has changed enormously.

On September 11, 2008, Charla had a heart transplant:

I almost died from not taking care of myself and I am so thankful that I finally figured things out before it was too late. I don't want others to do what I did or go through the pain I went through. I learned that a lot of the things I believed about myself weren't true. It was worth the effort to take care of myself and I didn't have to do it perfectly for it to count. When I started having heart disease, it was pretty much, you change or you die. I wasn't ready to die, and I didn't want to live the rest of my life feeling like I felt. So, I chose to live and make the best out of my life that I could.

I sometimes regret that I almost had to die to really let go of all the things I used to believe. As I started lowering my blood sugars, I felt better and had more energy to do what I wanted to do and more energy to do everything that I needed to do to take care of myself. I got on the upward spiral. I found it easier to take care of myself than I thought it would be. I am happier and healthier (if you can believe that), and thank goodness, because I need that energy to do what I need to do. I have to remind myself of how far I've come sometimes when it seems like too much.

I think making a choice made a difference. I choose to feel better so I can do the things I want to do.

TIPS

■ Dr. Ann Goebel-Fabbri says focus on food choices rather than food restrictions. Don't expect perfection in diet compliance.

- Avoid emotional or judgmental labels for foods or eating behaviors. Do not categorize foods as *good* or *bad*, or say that a person is *good* or *bad* based on how or what they eat.
- Make exercise a part of your life, not just a method of calorie burning. Becoming involved in life-long recreational sports like hiking or tennis makes exercise more fun and can help remove the exercise obsession as it relates to diabetes management.
- In addition, keep talking. Isolating and discussing the stressors in your life may help to alleviate them. Talking with family members, loved ones, or seeking professional counseling is an option. If you or your loved one exhibits the signs of an eating disorder, don't be afraid to talk about it. Open discussions with health professionals, family members, friends, spouses, and so forth.
- Recovery is possible and it does happen, the body heals well and in ways we don't always understand.

Treatment

Dr. Goebel-Fabbri says that treatment of eating disorders for women with diabetes is not about increasing the fear factor, but about providing the patient with a platform to keep talking. Treatment has to incorporate diabetes treatment and emotional components.

- Educate women about healthier coping strategies.
- Find a nutritionist who understands diabetes and eating disorders.
- Incorporate psychological needs with a social worker/counselor.
- Seek treatment with an eating disorder expert. (Dr. Goebel-Fabbri said that it's really important for treaters to understand the allure of easy loss of weight with insulin omission.)
- Understand the risks.
- Establish flexible eating patterns, end food restriction, and end rigid dieting (reduce binge eating).

- Take an active role in treatment.
- Seek a multidisciplinary team.
- Set realistic goals, gradual increase in amount of blood glucose monitoring, insulin intake.
- Problem-solve hurdles (eg, insulin edema).
- Fine-tune insulin management with doctors.

Dr. Goebel-Fabbri said that we still don't know the best treatment strategies:

> *In the inpatient or day treatment eating disorder centers, there is a gap between eating disorder meal planning and meal planning for women with diabetes. In the initial stages of treating an eating disorder, women need to rely on the structure of a fixed meal plan. The two treatment teams really need to communicate quite frequently so that they are not giving mixed messages and the patient doesn't get lost in the shuffle.*

She believes that patients need specialty treatment care, embedded with their diabetes treatment team:

> *I try to work to bridge between various diabetes treaters and the patient herself, to try to convey what her fears and struggles are about, and what the impediments are to her optimizing her diabetes treatment because of fear of weight gain, because of her concerns of taking too much insulin initially, and her lack of readiness in that regard. We try to develop some kind of "taste approach" to get her to gradually increase her insulin and get her blood sugars under a healthy range, not make it a one-size-fits-all because the patient is not ready for that.*

A lot of Dr. Goebel-Fabbri's work also incorporates diabetes education around what eating disorders are about and what diabetes management is. She said that the messages have changed in diabetes education over time, "initially, there were 'good foods' and 'bad foods,' ways you were supposed to eat which, in my opinion, were totally unrealistic for most people, and they sort of applied this moral judgment around certain types of foods." Dr. Goebel-Fabbri said that these rigid ideas about food, and which ones were okay, cheating, and doing it wrong, "those kinds of old style concepts about food and diabetes really mirror some of the moral judgment [that] someone with an eating disorder has." She says, "women with diabetes and disordered eating are getting that internal message from two different sources. They are caught between a rock and a hard place."

A Different Approach

A researcher who studies the psychosocial aspects of diabetes thinks the numbers are skewed. She asks, "What woman do you know who isn't body conscious?" She said that for many years, the medical establishment was taking the control away from women over their own intake and satiety and prescribing it in a rigid way. "Modern technology has allowed for more flexibility with eating, but women with diabetes have a disregulation with the hormone that controls appetite." "When behavior is attributed to maladjustment, it's unfair," she says. "I believe the results can be not weight motivated but one, an adherence to regimen and two, self-management."

Her recommendations for women with type 2 diabetes:

> It's also changing for women with type 2 . . . In the past, it was treatment to failure paradigm for women with type 2 diabetes. When they were first diagnosed, we would start them on diet and exercise, and if they failed, we would put them on oral meds and if they failed that, we started them on an insulin regimen. All that's changing. When you tell many type 2 women you have to go on insulin, they say, "oh no, I'm going to gain weight." She says there are modern discoveries, enhancements in treatments that are coming down the pipe that are going to make diabetes easier to take care of. The way we are asking you to eat is really no different than anybody else. (Eating moderately, exercising, etc.) You make life choices. It's about lifestyle, it's about how we eat.

PSYCHOLOGIST TIPS

■ Women need to be able to balance a sense of bodily integrity in the face of having a disease where one can't rely on one's cues.

■ When is it insulin omission and when is it insulin titration? (self-regulation)

■ A physician has only so much time to work with patients, and most are not managed by a team.

■ Reasons to be hopeful:

The true prevalence of eating disorders is probably some-what elevated from the general population, just because of what patients with diabetes have to live with on a daily basis. I think as we, healthcare providers, become more sophisticated and sensitized, the way we approach treatment is going to change.

Treatment Centers

1. **Behavioral Diabetes Institute (BDI).** Offers disordered-eating support groups.

Making Peace with Food, Insulin, and Your Body:
Are you living with type 1 diabetes and struggling with
an eating disorder? People with type 1 diabetes are at a
higher risk for eating disorders that can range from
disordered eating to restricting or omitting insulin,
also called diabulimia. Partake in honest discussion and
learn strategies for preventing and overcoming these
problems.

BDI offers a variety of workshops such as Insulin Omission and Diabulimia, Binge Eating Alumni Group, and Tackling Binge Eating in Diabetes.

Dr. Liana Abascal of BDI said that eating disorders can become part of a woman's identity and that the two biggest challenges of seeking treatment are (1) insulin omission works for weight loss and (2) a woman's ambivalence about change. Dr. Abascal said that at BDI, they conduct

6-week support group workshops with educational components and behavioral treatment practices. "We ask the women, what's getting in the way of change?" In the BDI workshops, Dr. Abascal recommends:

- Identifying food triggers
- Finding alternatives to binge eating
- Creating accountability
- Setting realistic goals
- Replacing negative self-talk

"We try to get the women to be nicer to themselves," she says.[1]

2. **Park Nicollet Melrose Institute.** Park Nicollet, in St. Louis Park, Minnesota, offers a specialized program for women with diabetes. Eating disorders paired with diabetes can be a life-threatening combination. Diabetes researchers estimate people who have type 1 diabetes have twice the risk of developing an eating disorder.

Melrose Institute collaborates with International Diabetes Center at Park Nicollet to treat people struggling with the dual diagnosis of an eating disorder and type 1 diabetes.

Care teams include pediatric and adult endocrinologists, psychiatrist, psychologist, diabetes nurse educator, and diabetes nutrition educator. A care manager helps to coordinate treatment, keeps the communication consistent, and answers questions for patients and families.

To learn more or schedule an initial assessment, call 952-993-6200.

If you have questions about type 2 diabetes, visit the website at: http://www.parknicollet.com/Diabetes/.[2]

3. **Center for Hope of the Sierras.** At the Center for Hope of the Sierras, they recognize that the treatment of co-occurring diabetes and eating disorders requires a highly specialized approach. The staff will help patients to find the balance between appropriate insulin intake and slow, gradual weight restoration while closely monitoring the individual's progress. Their unique approach includes educating patients about their bodies and their diseases so that they can learn to regulate the amount of sugar and carbohydrates they're consuming. This way, patients find a balanced, healthy weight they can be happy with, without feeling compelled to abuse insulin.

The diabetes program accounts for the biology of co-occurring diabetes and eating disorders as well as the psychological, social, and cultural implications that are interwoven in to the biological process. With treatment anchored in the biopsychosocial model, women in the diabetes program receive:

- Comprehensive medical management, including nutritional education and rehabilitation, blood sugar monitoring/testing, insulin administration, and a monitored exercise program
- Individual, group, and family therapy, which address the food, weight, body image, and interpersonal issues underlying an eating disorder, as well as the emotional factors that are interfering with responsible self-care for the treatment of diabetes.
- A home-like environment with 24-hour nursing and social support where women can connect in a meaningful way with peers, staff, and themselves.
- Comprehensive care from a team of experts in a Commission on Accreditation of Rehabilitation Facilities (CARF)-accredited residential program, including a board-certified pediatric endocrinologist, a registered dietician with a PhD in nutritional biochemistry, licensed psychologists and marriage and family therapists, a psychiatrist, and 24-hour nursing and patient assistants.[3]

With treatment and medical stabilization, patients learn that constant feelings of irritability, dehydration, and fatigue are not "normal" and that they can feel better when managing their diabetes in a healthy way. Patients learn better ways to cope with the feelings brought on by weight gain; they get educated about nutrition, diabetes management, and healthy living; and develop a support network that understands the implications of this dual diagnosis.

There are reasons to be hopeful. For example, women learn to eat in a way that adequately nourishes their bodies daily and preventively for future needs and challenges (i.e., growth, pregnancy, illness, aging). One psychologist's mantra is, "a balanced, moderate lifestyle, the same kind we would prescribe to anyone without diabetes." And finally, every woman should know that the progression of complications can be halted with treatment.

AUTHENTIC ADVICE

■ Lee Ann Thill says:

If girls today can find those few centers that treat diabetes and eating disorders, then they have a chance at recovery. However, a lot of hurdles still exist for women seeking treatment. A very important resource is Diabetes Moms. *The women who can teach their daughters about healthy eating and can impart a feeling of worth to their daughters.*

■ Charla says:

I've found good doctors who extend themselves more to me, knowing that I'm trying. I also volunteer with BDI. If I had at 15 years old what I have now, my life would have been so different. I want to tell people it can be different, it doesn't have to be this way. All I can do is tell you what I did, without judgment. We continue to struggle but we do have hope.

5   Exercise

One of the first questions I asked my doctor when I was diagnosed with type 1 diabetes at 14 years old was, "Will I still be able to play sports?" Six weeks into my fall semester at boarding school in New Hampshire, I was a proud member of the junior varsity field hockey team. I'd never been much of an athlete, which came as a surprise and a disappointment to my sports-loving mother who always told the story of when I was in the fourth grade and refused to join the soccer team at school. She was stunned. By the time I went away to school, I was ready to give sports another try. I liked the green and white kilts the girls on the field hockey team wore and the way they braided their hair down their backs and ran gracefully, holding the wooden stick in front of them as they chased the white ball across the field. So I joined the team and wore the kilt for 6 weeks, and then I got sick.

I was so sick that I skipped practice and went to the health center. The nurse gave me Tylenol and sent me back to the field where I lay on the green grass and listened to my teammates cheering on one another. Too tired to get up off the grass, I stared at the orange jug of water, desperately licking the dry roof of my mouth.

"Yes of course," my doctor said. "Diabetes won't keep you from doing any of the things your friends can do. Exercise is very important for people with diabetes, whenever your sugar [level] is high, go for a walk or a run." I remember feeling disappointed with his prescription for a healthy diet, consistent exercise, and daily regimen of insulin. It was anticlimactic. In my head, "disease" meant staying in bed in a room with the shades closed. I'd seen what people looked like with illness in *General Hospital*, and the picture my doctor was painting didn't match. I think I wanted to know how I was going to be different from then on. I wanted to know how my classmates were going to tell that I was someone with a chronic illness. "They won't," my doctor and parents told me, urging me back out onto the field.

Back at school, in an attempt to control my blood sugar levels, I started running. I'd always hated to run. I'd begun on the field hockey season, cutting through the woods during our daily runs with my friend Trish. She and I lingered in the back of the group, and when the coach wasn't looking, we took a shortcut. Walking under the trees, we cut the distance in half and rejoined our team as they neared the field. The coach never knew a thing, or so we thought. At the end of our season, my coach gave joke awards. I still have mine; it's a cardboard cutout of a foot in a running shoe that reads, "Most Unlikely Runner." She told the story of how shocked she'd been when she saw me running by her front porch on a Sunday, our day off. "The last girl I thought I'd see running when she didn't have to," she laughed and I was embarrassed but proud.

My coach didn't know why I was running and I never told her. When my blood sugar was high, I went for a run. When it was "normal," that meant I could eat something before I ran, something that wasn't in my "diabetes meal plan," something like a blueberry muffin or a glass of chocolate milk, and I ran the sugar out of my body. I kept running in college, along the trails that wandered up into the mountains at the University of Colorado; and when I graduated, I began to enter races. I learned to wake up early, give myself a shot, and eat breakfast at least an hour before the race began. Some runs were great, and other times I struggled, pushing myself up over the Cooper River Bridge 10K when my blood sugar was high. My legs strained, I was thirsty and just wanted to rest for a moment. But I kept going.

I kept going and eventually trained for a marathon. Searching for books about diabetes and marathons, I grew frustrated. I found books suggesting brisk walks, but there was nothing about running a marathon. I realized I would have to learn from my mistakes. And I made so many mistakes. After getting low on a training run, I learned to place bottles of Gatorade along the route and stop at the 10-mile mark that circled back to where my car was parked, and then I tested my blood sugar. Empty bottles of Gatorade filled the backseat of my car as a kind of trophy, like the blisters on my feet and the hardened muscles in my legs. I ran with a friend and carried jelly beans in my running shorts. I trained with a Team in Training group raising money for leukemia. After 4 months of training, I flew to Walt Disney World with my team.

The night before the race, I ate a big bowl of pasta for dinner to carbo-load. I woke up in the middle of the night to test my blood sugar and discovered I was low. I drank orange juice and ate a granola bar, and when the alarm went off at 5 a.m., my blood sugar was 260. I took a shot and ate a small bowl of cereal, wanting to stick to my routine. My teammates and I got on the bus and headed for the starting line. As I stood in the pack of runners covering their bodies with Vaseline and bending head over heels to stretch, I could tell that my blood sugar was high. The gun went off; I took a deep breath and started running. The first few miles passed by quickly because of the adrenalin, but by mile 7, my high blood sugar was wearing me down. My plan was to test my blood sugar before and after the race, so I didn't have to carry any equipment with me (this was before the days of continuous glucose monitoring (CGM), although I don't wear one even now). The sun had come up and was hot as we ran around a track, and I was struggling. By mile 12, my blood sugar finally began to drop and I could breathe again. I ran smoothly until I hit the wall at mile 22. I stopped to walk and eat a power bar. Limping along for the last 2.5 miles, I kept my eyes peeled for the finish line. As I passed through the gate after 4 ½ hours of running, I had never been so glad to stop moving.

I know I'd do a better job if I ran a marathon today because of what I learned that first time around. At 40 years old, I run every morning, pushing the baby jogger while my son Reid chatters happily to the passersby. I run because when I do, I enter a state of calm where my worries disappear with the rhythmic pounding of my feet. It's no longer about getting to eat forbidden foods, it's about taking care of my body. I run faster along the trail, and with the wind at my back, I feel ageless and strong. When I'm running, I don't feel like I have a disease.

The cardboard running shoe is at the bottom of a box in our shed marked "High School." When my coach handed me the joke award in front of my teammates so many years ago, I was embarrassed but proud. I have diabetes and I am a runner.

BENEFITS OF EXERCISE

- Increased self-confidence
- Reduced risk of heart disease
- Weight loss
- Lowered blood pressure

- Improved immune system
- Increased psychological well-being (release of endorphins)
- Stress release
- Improved muscle strength, bone density, and oxygen utilization

Cheryl Alkon has had "proliferative retinopathy" for approximately 10 years. She's had five laser treatments for it while pregnant. Proliferative retinopathy is the fourth stage of diabetic retinopathy where an abnormal growth of blood vessels occurs. By themselves, these blood vessels do not cause symptoms or vision loss. However, they have thin, fragile walls. If they leak blood, severe vision loss and even blindness can result.[1]

I have never had a vision problem, and don't even wear glasses. Regardless, my eye doctor told me that I shouldn't "lift anything over 15 pounds" or do "exercise that is jarring." As I have lifted heavy weights at assorted times in my life, was really getting into jogging the summer I did two triathlons, and actually felt better than ever, I was frank with the doctor about wanting to see specific research telling me that I should stop exercising hard, which she couldn't provide. I got my endocrinologist involved in the e-mail exchange, and pretty much decided that, until I am actively bleeding from my eyes, I will not curtail any hard exercise (i.e., lifting heavy weights, running, or even lifting my now 36-pound son to hug him) ever.

Judith Jones Ambrosini thinks the magic word to diabetes management is *exercise*.

First of all, I am in full agreement with the "Exercise is Medicine" movement formulated a couple years ago. I have always been physically active yet never competitive, except with myself. I truly enjoy movement, my favorites being dance and distance walking. I take jazz/aerobic and any other dance classes I can find. I do a 15-mile walk every Sunday morning and have walked a couple

*marathons; my favorite was the Copenhagen-Malmo
(Denmark-Sweden) a few years ago. I also use my bike for
transportation and have been studying tai chi for over
6 years. I teach tai chi exercises at a number of diabetes
conferences. The greatest reward for me is keeping everything in balance. Exercise plays a major part in living
with diabetes. Being outdoors for a walk or bike ride or
swim or any physical activity is invigorating and
motivating.*

QUESTIONS AND ANSWERS WITH DR. COLBERG-OCHS

Dr. Sheri Colberg-Ochs is an exercise physiologist, an author, a researcher,
and a professor of exercise science at Old Dominion University in
Virginia, who has written extensively about living with diabetes. She
was diagnosed with diabetes when she was 4 years old. Sheri says her
mom kept trying to "cure" her with alternative treatments, and when her
parents got divorced, her dad didn't want her to live with him because of
her diabetes.

*As a kid, I believed there was something wrong with me;
and as long as I have this disease, there will always be
something wrong with me. It took me a long time to get
over that and not feel like I was diseased and that I wasn't
worthy of being loved just the way I was, but it's just who
you are, it's part of you, you didn't ask for it, you didn't
deserve it, but everybody has something to deal with in
life. If they don't have it now, they'll have it later—it's just
the way it is.*

**What is the key to keeping blood sugar levels normal during
exercise?**

Plan ahead. What you're trying to do is replicate what the body normally
does doing exercise. One key to focus on is to try to moderate the circu-
lating levels of insulin (lower basal rate before you start, cut back on
basal doses, correct with carbs-glucose tabs, don't over-treat!). Use a

quick-acting source of carbs, such as candy or glucose tabs, and then a balanced amount of carbs, fat, and protein. "I used glucose tabs today when I was swimming," Sheri laughs, "even [though] I don't get it right all the time. It's sort of an art form, no one gets it right all the time, especially with women, and there's a huge effect with the monthly hormone cycle, it's just the way it is. There's just some days when you scratch you're head. Don't hold it against yourself. What I've learned in my 42 years of diabetes is that you don't need to whack yourself over the head. Live life first and be diabetic second. There's no guilt, because that doesn't help."

Is there a type of exercise that is best for women with diabetes?

What I recommend for everybody is if they only have time for one exercise, I would add resistance training.

Why does my blood sugar sometimes go up when I exercise?

Although moderate aerobic workouts usually cause your blood sugars to decrease while you're doing them, anaerobic or other intense work can cause them to rise instead due to an exaggerated release of glucose-raising hormones. However, even if a workout raises your blood glucose level temporarily, over a longer period of time (2–3 hours), the residual effects of the exercise will bring your blood sugar back down while replacing the carbs in your muscles. Intense work uses muscle glycogen faster, which can help keep your insulin action higher over the following day or two.

What about injuries, are we more prone to injuries as women with diabetes (foot care)?

We do have bigger risks for joint and overuse injuries. One way you prevent these injuries is by not doing the same thing every day. Common injuries are adhesive capsulitis ("frozen shoulder"), carpal tunnel syndrome (wrist pain), metatarsal fractures (of the foot bones), and neuropathy-related joint disorders (e.g., Charcot foot) in people with peripheral neuropathy. Additionally, people who have had diabetes for a long time are prone to nerve compression syndromes at the elbow and wrist that may be aggravated by repetitive activities, prolonged gripping, or direct nerve compression during weight training, cycling, and other activities. In most cases, good control of your blood sugar levels can reduce your risk of developing these injuries.

How does exercise increase insulin sensitivity?

The biggest way to maximize your insulin potential is with physical activity. There is a limited storage capacity in your body for carbs, and most get stored in your skeletal muscle. Once those carb storages are filled up and you eat more carbs, they don't have anywhere to go-there is a limited capacity. The more muscle mass you have, the greater storage capacity is for carbs; the more carbs you can store in your muscle, the shorter carbs will stay in your bloodstream after you eat them. When your muscles are full with carbs, that's one of the things that makes you insulin resistant; but your fat cells are not, so those carbs get converted into fat. That muscle mass is critical, otherwise you have to cut way back on the amount of carbs you eat.

What do you think about "carbo-loading" the night before a race?

It simply comes down to how the body works, and using carbs is more fuel efficient. Carbs are like using a higher-octane fuel, resulting in more miles to the gallon. If you want to exercise intensely and you eat a low-carb diet, you will simply not be able to perform at the highest level possible. However, if you're eating enough calories to cover your body's basal needs and your exercise use, you can easily get by with 40 percent or less of your calories coming from carbs. Eating more carbs than that will not necessarily benefit exercise (it is *not* a case of "some is good, so more is better"). I do believe that most people who are training overdo their carb intake, given the limited amount and intensity of training that they do. For example, you really don't need to eat a huge pasta dinner the night before you do a 5K (3.1 miles) run.

Tell me about "erasing your mistakes."

In her book, *50 Secrets of the Longest Living People with Diabetes* (2008), Sheri talks about "Erasing Your Mistakes." She writes about "erasing" blood sugar mistakes with exercise:

> *Although your muscles account for only about 40 percent of your body weight, they can take up 80 percent of any*

glucose load that you get through your carbohydrate intake. Thus, by enhancing your muscles' capacity to take up glucose with or without insulin, exercise comes closer than anything else to "erasing" your mistakes with your food, insulin, or other medications that lead to hyperglycemia . . . . During this time, you will likely need considerably less insulin to process any carbohydrates that you eat, and you can get away with eating more carbs after exercise, particularly if it was strenuous and prolonged.[2]

What should I eat postexercise?

Chocolate milk and low-carb yogurt work well, as do soy milk, ice cream (preferably low sugar), and other carb/protein/fat-balanced foods. Actually, in the diabetes world, we have known for quite some time that whole milk postexercise helps keep blood glucose levels more stable and prevent late-onset hypoglycemia than sports drinks, skim milk, or water, but it's good to know that our postexercise secret has now spread to the rest of the world as an exercise recovery aid!

TIPS

- Plan ahead.
- Cross-train, don't do the same thing every day.
- If you only have time for one exercise, do resistance training— the biggest way to maximize insulin potential is through exercise.
- Alternate hard and easy days; harder days will help with blood sugar control for approximately 2 days, so space the hard and easy days out.

Sheri's personal exercise routine is based on alternating easy and hard days:

Monday: gym, cardio, 30- to 45-minute resistance training, low sets with various activity
Tuesday: gym, moderate 30-minute bike ride, medium pace
Wednesday: swim 1 hour
Thursday: moderate 30-minute exercise, medium pace

Friday: gym, cardio 30-minute resistance training, low sets with various activity
Saturday and Sunday: walk with husband, anywhere from 1 to 3 hours

"Every day I try to be as active as possible. I walk the stairs at work. That daily movement is really critical."

Sheri says people ask her all the time how she manages to balance work, family, exercise, and diabetes—and her answer is, "I exercise. That's the answer. If I didn't, I wouldn't have the endurance to do all the other things," she laughs. Sheri says she's never let diabetes keep her from doing anything she wanted to do, "Don't use diabetes as an excuse not to exercise, use it as an excuse *to* exercise!"

BALANCING BLOOD SUGAR LEVELS WITH EXERCISE

Mari Ruddy, a triathlete and founder of the Red Rider Recognition Program and Team WILD (Women Inspiring Life with Diabetes), says, "It's not really about blood sugar management, it's about insulin management, which ideally results in good blood sugar management."

As a child, Mari watched her athlete father struggle with managing his type 1 diabetes with very little knowledge or support from the world. He was regularly taken to the hospital with extreme low blood sugar issues. These incidents almost always coincided with exercise, whether planned or spontaneous. From her eyes as a child, it seemed that no matter what her father did to be proactive, things went wrong and she feared for her father's life. As a result, when Mari was diagnosed with type 1 diabetes at age 16, she was afraid to push her body to the limit for fear of suffering deathly consequences.

> *This led to poorly controlled diabetes until I was 35, when I finally found an endocrinologist and a coach who worked together to walk me through my fears. They provided intensive support and education about how I could exercise and manage my diabetes successfully. It turns out that exercise and movement is a key to living well in general and with diabetes in particular. . . . What I know in my heart is that every woman alive who sets her body, heart, and mind to it is an athlete. I want to help her figure out how to take it from an idea to an everyday reality. Diabetes can be an opportunity to learn about oneself.*

Ann Rosenquist Fee says timing is the tricky part:

The other night, I asked my son if he wanted to play racquetball at the Y, and he said yes, so when we had dinner, I ate without taking any short-acting insulin first. When we were ready to leave, I called the Y to reserve a court, but the receptionist said all the courts were booked for a handball tournament.

For my son, no big deal, he could live without racquetball that night. For me, though, it was the big deal that drives my exercise practice: I'd loaded up on carbs without any NovoLog, so I had to get moving whether the courts were open or not, or else spend the night sitting around in the 200s looking forward to a shitty A1c.

I went to the Y by myself and did 30 minutes on the elliptical, which is what I usually do a few nights a week at the right time after the right amount of carbs. Or I walk the trails in our town, or bike, or I use my weighted Hula-Hoops in the basement. It's nice when the timing works out to play with my kid, or walk with my husband or a friend, but diabetes trumps having an exercise partner.

Or maybe diabetes is my exercise partner. Even if the racquetball courts are closed, or my husband decides he's too "in-his-slippers-already" for the Y, or my friend who walks the neighborhood after dark decides she's staying in that night, my untreated 200 mg/dl is still there, urging me on.

I should think about it like that. Like a partner. A blood-sugar-shaped coach. Skinny and rude like a syringe, with little syringe-cap-orange sweatbands and leg warmers. Barking her mean little bark like, "I don't care that the courts are closed. You're above 200. Get out the door. Get moving. Keep moving. And I'll see you after dinner tomorrow."

Melinda Law has had type 1 diabetes for 50 years, and exercise has been an integral part of her life. She says:

I go to the gym 2–3 days a week, at 5–6 a.m. I do aerobics for 30 minutes, either the stair climber, bicycle, or

*treadmill, and then I do weights and machines for 30 min-
utes and make sure I work up a sweat. It's a lot of fine-
tuning, but I have my basal down to 0.50 per hour. The
glycogen gets released 2 hours later so my basal is up to
0.60 2 hours later for 2 hours, then back down. The other
2 days I take off the pump and swim, and am in the pool
for 45 minutes. It always makes me feel better. As soon as I
start doing anything, I feel freedom, whether it's
ice-skating, motocross, skiing, swimming, running, road
racing, trampoline, bicycling, or any other physical
activity. For a long time, I was very discouraged because I
could not figure out how to exercise without having my
numbers go too low. I was constantly asking and just
started slowly but surely figuring it out. I always test before
and after. Always.*

*As a kid, there wasn't anything I did not do. I ran, played
baseball, basketball, football, volleyball, punchball, stick-
ball, tennis, horseback riding, swimming, water skiing,
sailing, biking, you name it, I did it. I taught horseback
riding and jumping and was on the team in college. Skiing
got me through law school, since I went every other
weekend. The funny thing is, I see myself as uncoordinated
and gawky, not athletic at all. I love to use my body, but
don't see myself as an athlete. It was drilled into my head
at a very young age to exercise every day to bring down
blood sugar. I was outside running around as a kid, for
3 hours a day no matter what.*

Annie Berger, who played Division 1 soccer in college, says that
when she's doing something intense, she will test her blood sugar level
before, during, and after exercise.

*I've learned that there are certain activities that make
me drop quickly, some that make my drop hours afterwards, and some, such as competitive sports, that actually cause me to go very high because of all the
adrenaline. Depending on the activity, I will often eat at
some point, whether it is right before, in the middle of, or
after exercising.*

Getting Low While Exercising

Getting low while exercising happens to everyone at some time or another. I remember running on a treadmill in the gym one summer when it was too hot to run outside. My kids were unhappy in the Kids' Club there. I promised them that we would only stay for 1 hour and I knew they were looking at the clock. This was my only chance to run. But I could feel my blood sugar dropping, and I had to stop mid-run to prick my finger. I was 40. Determined to get some exercise, I pulled out my bag of Skittles and ran while I chewed, all the while trying not to fall off. Was it worth it? I'm not sure. It wasn't the first time I've had to eat on the run and it won't be the last.

Melinda Law says:

> *When I exercise, I always, always, always carry something with me. At the gym and swimming it is easy because I throw GU gel or the little chewy things in my bag. When I run, I usually put them in my shorts pocket.*

Lesley Hoffman Goldenberg always has a tube of glucose tablets with her.

> *I place them on the machine when I work out. If I go for a walk in the park, I always bring a little wristlet or an equally cool (or uncool) fanny-pack-type thing to hold all of my diabetes goodies.*

Judith Jones Ambrosini never leaves the house without her number one favorite sugar fix, the classic candy Chuckles.

> *Each Chuckle contains 9 carbs. The packet comes in five flavors: wild cherry is my favorite. Two of these candies taste great and usually do the trick of bringing up a low by 40 points. One pack of Chuckles fits nicely in any pocket. I don't like to carry things, so pockets are always a priority for me when buying clothes.*

Managing Diabetes During Competitions

Cheryl Alkon says that when she was training for a triathlon, she was upfront with her coaches about diabetes.

They told me they'd do what they could, but had only worked with type 2s before. I was always on top of things (i.e., I always had the juice box on me if needed), and nothing ever happened during that training period (i.e., no blackouts, no terrible lows I couldn't handle, etc.) At the end of the training period, they actually singled me and another woman out (a cancer survivor) for an award for training with additional health challenges, and I had mixed feelings about it. My first thought was, "Oh, really?" I managed everything just fine. I don't need a special mention for that! But after talking about it with a therapist I was working with at the time (also [with] type 1 [diabetes]), she said, "Actually, that was pretty impressive that they recognized what you were dealing with. You shouldn't discount it," which I suppose is true, but overall, I feel like I manage things pretty well every day, and I don't really see anyone giving me an award for that. It's just the way I live my life.

Jennifer Ahn, member of Team WILD, says:

It's a great way of sharing ideas and experience [about] diabetes with exercise together. On the training groups that are not diabetes related, I do tell the coach and teammates about my diabetes so they are aware if I have issues with my blood sugars.

Annie Berger was a very athletic teen when she was first diagnosed.

One of my motivators to get out of the hospital was actually to go to a soccer tournament. My coach of that team was a doctor, so he handled it well. I don't remember telling my teammates, I think my coach must have done that. I think people reacted well because they went off of how I acted. They were of course concerned for me and always helped if I went low, but no one treated me that differently. I remember my high school soccer coach being scared at first and not knowing how to handle it, but we figured out together how it affected me and both learned quickly that it didn't need to be a big deal. That coach was also my high school lacrosse coach, so that made things easy. I think my college soccer coach was intimidated by my having diabetes. I think she thought I couldn't handle playing in games. When I played more and more in my sophomore year, she saw that I could handle it just fine. It was a learning process, but she learned how to handle it. I've never had issues with any of my teammates. They were always very supportive.

Seeking Motivation

Kathleen Fraser was invited to be the inspirational speaker at a camp for families affected by type 1 diabetes.

When they reached out to me, I thought, "Me, an inspirational speaker? What could I possibly say that would inspire parents and children with diabetes?"

The most poignant moment came at the end of my talk when a mom asked me my motivation for doing triathlons. Without hesitation I said, "Because I have diabetes and I can." It was so simple, the most natural response, and in my mind, it said it all. There was peace in the room and knowing looks on the faces of the parents. It was as if this hard, cold classroom filled with strangers was transformed into a warm, cozy living room with friends and family. They knew right then and there that all would be okay for them and their children. They were now in on the coveted secret: Diabetes doesn't have to stand in your way of accomplishing your goals and fulfilling your dreams.

Yes, having diabetes makes it harder, but in all honesty, not any harder than it is to live with diabetes each and every day. It's an integral part of who I am, and the challenges I face as a woman living with diabetes enable me to say with confidence that I am stronger and more resilient because of diabetes and because of my athletic journey with diabetes.

Through exercise, I have learned more about myself as an individual, a woman, and a person living with diabetes.

I now know that I can do anything. I no longer question if I can overcome a new challenge from a diabetes perspective. I have the knowledge and support to figure it out.

The journey to educate myself started with Team WILD (Women Inspiring Life with Diabetes). Through Team WILD, I was able to get the information I needed about what it takes to be an active and healthy person. Before Team WILD, I looked at myself as a person with diabetes first and a human being second. Now I know what nutrition my body needs to stay active and fit, first and foremost. Through the support and education of WILD coaches, medical staff, and teammates, I can not only swim, bike, and run safely and successfully but I can also hike, do yoga, Pilates, and even take long, leisurely walks in the park with confidence and security.

Having more diabetes management tools in my toolbox gives me the confidence to be fully engaged in life. I do triathlons because I have diabetes. I get out there every day and exercise because I want to be stronger and more in touch with my body. I feel empowered and powerful.

Linda Frick enjoys walking a few miles on the beach every Sunday with her husband and friends.

I also belong to a gym and walk on the treadmill for 30 minutes and then work the resistance machines for another 30 minutes. I try to go twice a week, but often, my fatigue gets in the way.

Sadly, I have to say that I have never been motivated to exercise. I was 8 when I was diagnosed and, of course, it was easy to get daily exercise at that age. I was not interested in sports as a child, so did not compete in any organized youth sports. As an adult, the only thing that motivates me is my own vanity (yes, that's what I said—vanity!). Diabetes does not motivate me to work out and sweat. My appearance, how my clothes fit,

*and how I feel do motivate me however. My body metab-
olism slowed way down when I turned 50 and, ever
since, exercise is a must in order to keep my weight
under control.*

Andie Dominick, author of *Needles*, says one of the reasons she is
such an avid exerciser is because of her diabetes.

*I believe it has helped me maintain good circulation and
blood sugar control after 30 years of type 1 diabetes. I
rode RAGBRAI (bike ride across Iowa, about 500 miles)
seven times. Two years ago, I walked a 26-mile marathon.
I walk on the weekends with friends instead of going out
to eat or have drinks. Most of my family's activities are
centered around exercise. In fact, if we want to go to
dinner, we walk there. The neighbors joke about seeing us
walk everywhere.*

Challenges to Exercising

Linda Frick's biggest challenge is energy level and age.

*There is not enough time to work out prior to going to
work and when I get home at the end of my day, I'm tired
and just want to relax and enjoy my home and family. So
I have to stay focused on my appearance as my reason for
pushing myself. It does seem to work for me. I've invested
lots of money in clothes for my job and if they don't fit, I'm
in big trouble. It's either starve or work out and I usually
choose the latter.*

Lesley Hoffman Goldenberg says being spontaneous is a challenge.

*I work 30 blocks from where I live, which is about a mile
and a half. If it's nice out and I have some time to kill, I love
taking a brisk walk home because it's a great way to end
my day. Unfortunately, I can't make the decision right when
I leave work like most people. I have to start planning in the
afternoon because I could need a snack, set a temporary
basal, or not walk at all because my sugar is too high, and*

I'd have to stop to use the bathroom every few blocks. I hate that spontaneity cannot be a part of diabetes. It's good because I'm a big planner, but it gets annoying sometimes.

I also find it challenging to check my sugar if I'm using a cardio machine that involves my whole body. Usually, I can balance and it totally works out, and I've got it down to a science. But with certain machines, I lose my balance or drop a testing strip (at a $1 per strip) and I just get frustrated.

EXERCISE AND MENTAL HEALTH BENEFITS

When I go for a run, I almost always return home in a good mood. When I'm out on the trail and breathing steadily, my mind begins to drift and, suddenly, those things that were driving me crazy before I left the house (the kids, the house, the bills, the work, etc.) don't seem like such a big deal. People call it "runner's high" and, scientifically, we know that endorphins are released through exercise.

On her website, Sheri Colberg-Ochs writes about exercise and the benefits to emotional health. She says, "A good reason to try to enhance and uplift your mood is the very well documented, but poorly understood, mind–body connection. Physical health and mental health are undeniably interrelated, and each affects the other; accordingly, your physical well-being often can't be improved if your psychological problems haven't been adequately addressed. Depression is an illness affecting both your mind and your body. When in a depressed state, you may feel sluggish, lethargic, apathetic toward your self-care, or downright uninterested in everything. Is it any wonder that it's difficult to manage your diabetes and stay healthy when you're depressed?"[3]

Everyone—people with and without chronic health conditions—can use regular exercise to relieve mild-to-moderate symptoms of depression and anxiety, as well as to improve mood and self-perceptions. If you're physically active, particularly if you're a woman (which already makes you more prone to depression than a man), you'll experience better mental and physical health and less depression than someone who is physically inactive.

Exercise is the best "medicine." As I mentioned previously, becoming physically active can also positively affect your self-perceptions, benefiting your self-confidence, self-concept, and self-esteem. Especially for women and girls, dissatisfaction with our bodies is associated with lower self-esteem. If you perceive yourself as fat and out of shape, you'll be particularly vulnerable to a negative self-image. We're all more and more susceptible to such bodily misperceptions because of the media. For instance, overweight teens who spend more time watching soap operas, movies, music videos, and sports reportedly have an even greater bodily dissatisfaction and drive for thinness than those who don't. Exercise acts as "medicine" because it can improve your body shape and size and, consequently, raise your self-esteem and improve your bodily satisfaction, particularly if you're overweight. Not only can exercise improve your short-term mental state and mood, but you can also use it to increase your overall sense of well-being over the long haul.

EXERCISE AND TYPE 2 DIABETES

Exercise is very important in managing type 2 diabetes. Combining diet, exercise, and medicine (when prescribed) will help control your weight and blood sugar level. In her book, *The Diabetic Athlete*, Sheri Colberg-Ochs says, "Exercise can be a vital component in the prevention and management of type 2 diabetes when used in conjunction with diet, oral medications, and insulin therapies" (p. 79).[4]

Kelly Love Johnson was diagnosed with type 2 diabetes in her 30s. She says:

> *When I was initially diagnosed, it was difficult because I worked so much. I joined a gym that had TVs on their treadmills and made it a priority. I figured I had time to watch TV in the evenings, so I may as well walk while I did it! One of my tricks is that I'd try to get to the gym before one of my favorite shows started. I walked at a fairly fast pace during the show and sprinted (at 5.5) during commercials. Sprints are a great way to burn fat, and if I knew I only had to do them during commercials, it was like a carrot on a stick for me. Did I mention that I hate to exercise? I'm not a gym person, so when my membership expired, I looked for other ways to get cardio, bought a bicycle, and had a great time bicycling around my neighborhood. At the end of 2008, when I*

*found myself working from home again, I got a super
active puppy so I would be forced to get out of bed in the
morning and exercise first thing. I still walk (with the
dog) between 2.5 and 5 miles a day, but the great thing
about where I live now is that it's a hilly area, so even
just walking (especially up those hills) is good cardio
for me.*

I began running to control my blood sugar levels and I am still
running 25 years later because it makes me feel strong. When I was diagnosed, I had a doctor who gave me a positive first impression of living
with diabetes. I'm thankful because he gave me a prescription to live a
healthy life. Running became a tool to manage my health. When my
blood sugar levels were high, I knew there was something (other than
the dreaded shot) I could do to help myself feel better. I have diabetes
and I am a runner.

AUTHENTIC ADVICE

■ Andie Dominick says:
*You have to make a point to exercise every day. Not three times
a week. Not on the weekends. Every day. That doesn't just
mean taking the stairs. It means making a point to exercise. And
everyone has time. Instead of "relaxing" in front of the television
for an hour or two at night, set up a treadmill in the living room
and watch while you walk or jog. Get out of the car and walk
around the neighborhood. Most of us sit all day in our jobs. We
shouldn't be sitting when we're off the clock. The human body
craves movement.*

■ Cheryl Alkon says:
*I met with an exercise physiologist at the recommendation of
my endo[crinologist] before I started the tri[athlon] training, and
while he had some general advice for a type 1, it all boiled
down to "use trial and error to figure out how things work for*

you," which, while frustrating, is what I'd tell someone else. I have a lot of pregnancy weight I need to lose, and that excess weight affects how much insulin [I need] to take for correction factors, and other things. It's really different from person to person.

■ Mari Ruddy says:

I love setting goals and I love having a reason, beyond managing diabetes, to write everything down: food, sleep, blood sugars, insulin, stress levels, what I do for exercise. High-level athletes all record this information, and being in their company helps me stay strong with good diabetes management, which ends up [from] being a fabulous by-product to being an endurance athlete.

■ Rachel Garlinghouse says:

Find what makes you happy. I, for example, hate running. I attempted several times to start a running routine, only to find that I still hated running. So instead, I walk (which I enjoy), I lift weights, and I clean my house on days when I don't want to go to the gym but still need to break a sweat to keep my sugars under control. There are so many different ways to get a good workout. There's gardening, there's playing on a team, there's dancing, there's classes at the gym. Whatever you do, don't just do nothing.

■ Linda Frick says:

It will be extremely hard for someone to start a fitness routine that is not used to it, but the payoff will be that you feel so much better. It will give you more energy and will also give you self-esteem about yourself. You have to see past the first 20 minutes of any exercise regimen and then you are on the homestretch. Take brisk walks in a place that you like (mine happens to be [at] the beach with its wonderful sounds and smells). Make it fun and enjoyable, and know that sometimes you won't feel like it, but the rewards will be great. If you belong to a gym, invest in a trainer so that you will know how to use the equipment and can track your progress. Whatever you decide to do, do it for yourself.

■ Kelly Love Johnson says:

Find something you enjoy doing, even if you have to try 20 different things before you hit on the right one. Change up your routine. I can't "just" do yoga or "just" walk because boredom will set in. I take different types of yoga classes, hit different walking trails, love my Sketchers Shape-Ups, go roller-skating every now and then, and still ride my bike occasionally. I'd love to take a kickboxing class next. I think if you change up your routine and find things you actually enjoy doing, even if you hate to exercise, you can still do it.

6   Dating, Sex, and Marriage

I fell in real love for the first time when I was 23. He was a tall, dark, and handsome Southern boy who called me *babe*. No one had ever called me babe before. I started dating him right around the time that I started working on getting my blood sugars tighter. The results of the Diabetes Control and Complications Trial (DDCT)—a major clinical study conducted from 1983 to 1993, funded by the National Institute of Diabetes and Digestive and Kidney Diseases, which showed how keeping blood glucose levels as close to normal as possible slowed the onset and progression of the eye, kidney, and nerve damage caused by diabetes—had just been released, and my endocrinologist was one of the doctors involved in the study. A recent college graduate, my endocrinologist encouraged me to test more and get my blood sugars tighter. It was the first time, since I was diagnosed, that I began to work hard to improve my health. I kept my blood sugar records and recorded my results on a daily basis and then brought my records to my endocrinologist to make adjustments. It was during this time that I met Jason.

I told Jason about my diabetes shortly after we met and I remember that he was kind and curious and that it was such a relief. It was the first time I was taking my health somewhat seriously and I was thrilled that he was there to support me. We'd been dating for about a month before we slept together. I remember that we spent the night at his apartment, but I don't remember waking up beside him. What I do remember is hearing the voices of his roommates—a girl and a guy—telling me that Jason would be back soon and everything would be okay. I remember thinking, "Please no, please no," and wanting to fall back asleep and return to the moment before my blood sugar dropped. Jason told me later that he'd woken up and I was lying next to him covered in sweat and unresponsive. My parents lived just a few blocks away and he'd run

123

to their house to ask for help, but no one was home. He then ran to my sister's apartment, and she told him to get me orange juice. He returned to the apartment with juice, picked me up, and poured the juice down my throat. As I began my slow return to the real world, I'd been ashamed and embarrassed, and knew that I'd said things I shouldn't have said. But Jason was smiling and holding me close, and putting his strong arms around me, he told me I was *cute* and that he liked *taking care of me*.

Everything changed from that day on. I realized that he'd seen the worst of me (or so I thought) and that he could handle it. He wasn't afraid and he even seemed to think that the worst of me was acceptable, loveable even. But it didn't last. I became obsessive about my blood sugars, keeping them tighter and tighter and having more and more lows. We were in love and it was really powerful, and it was really heartbreaking when it was over. I'm not sure how much of it had to do with diabetes; I realized eventually that we were not meant to be, but I always wondered how much my frequent lows had to do with his leaving. Looking back, I think that diabetes was just a part of the end of our relationship and that real love means someone who loves all of you, but it was a difficult life lesson and a bitter pill to swallow at 23 years old.

As women with diabetes, we can't walk away when things get rough. We are in this relationship with our bodies for the rest of our lives, and just like any other relationship, we have to nurture our physical selves. Having someone there beside you, to support you when things are good and when things are bad, makes this journey so much better. Having a partner who understands the physical and emotional demands of living with diabetes is a reward, and supportive relationships have been proven to result in improved diabetes management. But these relationships don't fall out of the sky, it takes work and communication to survive, so here are a few stories and tips on how to find and maintain a healthy sexual relationship.

RELATIONSHIP STATISTICS

A survey conducted by MicroMass Communications, based on findings from 828 women with type 1 and type 2 diabetes, found that:

- Almost half of women report that diabetes has a negative impact on their sex lives.
- 58 percent of those questioned did not know that the menstrual cycle can trigger changes in blood sugar.

- Along with diminished libido, 25 percent of the women who responded to the survey reported loss of spontaneity, and 22 percent said they were less likely to reach orgasm.
- Nearly three out of four of those questioned had trouble managing their weight, and nearly half had trouble choosing the right foods. Half of them reported that controlling their blood sugar was a major challenge, and one out of three admitted that they found it hard to take care of themselves before looking after others.[1]

Andi Kravitz Weiss, MPH, says:

Our research shows that women with diabetes have far more confidence in their ability to take their medications than they have in their ability to make basic lifestyle changes. As a result, health care providers should be providing education and support programs that help build that confidence so that women can learn how to make the lifestyle changes necessary to successfully manage their diabetes.

Weiss refers to this discrepancy as "the confidence gap."[1] She says the women who reported higher confidence in lifestyle management felt more sexually attractive. Some of these key findings follow:

- Approximately one-third of respondents felt diabetes had made an adverse impact in their desire for sex.
- 38 percent of respondents said that diabetes had a negative impact on their body image.
- 28 percent of respondents indicated that diabetes had a negative impact on their general happiness.

BUILDING THE CONFIDENCE TO LIVE WELL

Having knowledge is one thing, but confidence is the link between knowing what to do and actually doing it. Confidence plays a significant role in the successful management of diabetes. Women who feel confident in their ability to manage diabetes are less likely to blame themselves for having the disease, are less likely to worry about themselves, and are less likely to hide their condition from others. Additionally, they are more likely to experience a more satisfying sex life.

Confidence is not something that's necessarily innate. It requires education, practice, and support. Whereas 84 percent of survey respondents said they feel confident in their ability to take their diabetes medication as prescribed, less than half indicated that they had a level of certainty regarding the holistic management of their condition.

Four core behavioral strategies can be used to incorporate elements that build skills and confidence. They are:

- Involving women in their own care
- Using goal-setting techniques: Identifying what to work on to reduce the feeling of being overwhelmed
- Engaging women in active learning for skill building: Weiss suggests setting specific goals
- Exploring feelings and developing coping skills with support groups (such as DiabetesSisters and TuDiabetes)

Weiss says that many of the women in the survey who were under 45 years old reported being "too busy to take good care of themselves." She realized that in order to close this confidence gap, women with diabetes need to give themselves permission to take care of themselves, sometimes to put their needs first.

When to Talk About Diabetes With Your Date

Jennifer Ahn is fairly open with her diabetes when it comes to dating:

When I was dating, it would depend on how I met the person. I usually would let them know about my diabetes prior to meeting. If it was a blind date, however, I would refrain from telling them until it looked like it was going well. I met my current significant other (my fiancé) online. After exchanging a few emails, I shared with him my background, as we were planning our first date and going biking. I didn't want him to be alarmed if something happened during the ride. He appreciated my openness and asked some questions, that is, what to do if something did happen, how it affected me, and so forth. He asked whether it was the one I took pills for or insulin. It wasn't a big deal to me. It was nice to have it out in the open. There was no shame or embarrassment.

For Lesley Hoffman Goldenberg, sharing her secret was a little more uncomfortable:

When I first started dating my husband, I was so nervous to tell him I had diabetes. We got drinks and then dinner for our first date, and I ate the entire meal and then snuck into the bathroom to give myself insulin. Not a good idea—my sugar spiked up really high that night. For our second date, we went out to lunch and I did the same thing—ate two sushi rolls and took insulin like an hour later. I was on shots at the time, so it wasn't as easy as it is now with my pump. I decided to tell him on our third date. After discussing it with multiple friends and my mom for hours, I decided that straightforward, nonchalant, and simple was the way to go (ironically, those are three adjectives I would never, ever *use to describe diabetes). Anyway, we grabbed slices of pizza, and I said, "By the way, I have diabetes and I take insulin before I eat. It's totally not a big deal, just wanted you to know." (Ha, not a big deal!) He said something really nice and sensitive like, "Oh, okay, I have a coworker with diabetes so I know a little bit about it. Thanks for telling me."*

DIABETES IN THE BEDROOM

Ann Rosenquist Fee says that she has managed to keep diabetes out of the bedroom:

I was diagnosed just before my 3rd wedding anniversary. This summer, we'll celebrate our 25th. In those 17 years, diabetes has been less disruptive to my sex life than the

*glasses I wear at night, or the mouth guard I use to keep
from grinding my teeth when I sleep.*

*I don't wear an insulin pump, so as long as I can tell the
difference between the flush/sweat/rapid pulse of lust and
the flush/sweat/rapid pulse of hypoglycemia (I usually
can and in case not, I've got glucose tablets in a drawer
right next to the lube), diabetes stays out of my bed.*

How does a woman feel sexy with a plastic pump attached to her
legs, lower back, stomach, or arms? When your husband, boyfriend, or
girlfriend puts their hand around your back, how do you feel when they
brush against your pump? Do the bruises on your stomach from injections make you feel less desirable? Does the extra weight make you want
to dress in loose, less revealing clothing?

Having sex for the first time can be an exciting, embarrassing, and
overwhelming event. For young women with diabetes, the fact that we
have to think about our blood sugar and/or medical supplies getting in
the way can create additional feelings of self-consciousness. Diabetes
may keep some women from rushing into having sex, whereas diabetes
may act as a catalyst for others. For the rest, like Ann, diabetes won't
make a difference under the sheets at all.

Self-esteem and Sex

My personal theory is that in order to feel sexy and fully enjoy sex, we
need to feel pride instead of shame when it comes to our physical selves.
I think, many women with diabetes are often at war with their bodies.
We deny ourselves of food in order to be thin, beat ourselves up when
we eat more than we think we should, and when we look in the mirror,
we only see the things we don't like. As women with chronic illnesses,
we are constantly "battling" our bodies into submission, we are "waging
a war" against blood sugars, and war is not sexy. We treat our bodies like
scientific experiments, and our sexual satisfaction will only increase
when we learn to be kind to ourselves and honor our physical selves.
Having good sex and feeling sexy doesn't come naturally for a lot of
women, and if we want to get good at it, it'll take practice. We need to
learn to visualize our physical selves as healthy, strong, and sexy.

Research has shown that up to 35% of adult women with type 1 diabetes report sexual dysfunction. Dr. Albright says there is not a lot of

research about women, diabetes, and sexuality. "It appears as it is not as much about the complications or the blood sugar–blood pressure relationship that affects sexuality. It is shaped much more by confidence in yourself and by depression, and your relationship with your partner."

Lesley Hoffman Goldenberg says that there were a lot of other things to be self-conscious about, aside from wearing a pump.

Rachel Garlinghouse says that diabetes has taught her how important it is to take care of and be kind to her body:

> *I have curves and a healthy, able body. The most important thing is good health—not a number on the scale or a dress size. I appreciate how hard my body works for me, and I don't get caught up in insecurities, which will only hamper my diabetes progress. I have far too much going on in my life to stand in front of the mirror and pick out what I don't like about my body.*

Diabetes educator and type 1 diabetic Claire Blum says:

> *I believe it is important for women to know that decreased sex drive is not necessarily a part of having diabetes. There is conflicting evidence regarding the impact of blood glucose control and sex drive . . . but there are many variables in the research that have not been controlled for . . . including the variability of blood glucose (something we see mentioned a bit more now that people have CGM and are learning how to decrease that variability) . . . and there is evidence that improved glucose control is an important aspect of sexual health.*

> *The endocrinologist that I work with tells women that sexual interest and sex drive are a sign of health . . . which of course includes the integration of mind, body, soul . . . or balance. Good nutrition is an aspect of health that is often neglected with diabetes . . . with so much emphasis on taking the right amount of insulin and BG management . . . many women do not realize the importance of proper nutritional intake.*

> *This is one of the areas where I believe proper education and support is of utmost importance. Even though surveys and research may show that women with diabetes often*

experience a decrease in libido . . . it is important to recognize that a decrease in sexual desire is not an inherent outcome of diabetes. We can be as healthy, if not healthier, than woman who do not have diabetes. Sexual desire is a sign of health, and sensuality, a state of mind that is nurtured when we find balance in care of our body-mind-soul.

Understanding Our Bodies

Janis Roszler, RD, CDE, LD/N, the 2008–2009 Diabetes Educator of the Year (American Association of Diabetes Educators [AADE]), said that women need to understand their bodies. She has written several books about relationships and diabetes and gives talks to increase education about diabetes and sexuality.

Understanding the anatomy of our bodies includes more than knowing if we are high or low. We also need to know how our bodies work in order to achieve pleasure. Too many women think it is their fault when they can't achieve orgasm through sex with a partner, when in fact, statistics show that for all women, the percentage of achieving orgasm through plain, old-fashioned sex is low.

Part of understanding our body is understanding our menstrual cycle. Janis says arousal is affected for women with type 1 diabetes during the "luteal phase." From the day after ovulation until the day before the next period expect:

- Decreased arousal
- Impaired ability to achieve orgasm
- Increased discomfort/pain during sexual penetration
- Decreased sexual function independent of mood, not influenced by glycemic control

Orgasms are hard to achieve for many women, including women with diabetes. Rachel Garlinghouse says:

I know, without a doubt, that diabetes impacts every area of my life. If my sugars are too high, I'm dry all over, including vaginally. That's obviously not pleasant. If I'm low, sex isn't enjoyable. It's hard to be spontaneous when my number one priority has to be diabetes, not spur of the moment sex.

SEXUAL ISSUES FOR WOMEN

- Inability to achieve orgasm
- Decreased lubrication
- Pain/discomfort during intercourse
- Reduced libido
- Self-esteem (weight gain, injection/infusion set marks, etc.)

Causes:

- **Neuropathy.** Can affect ability to lubricate or experience orgasm
- **Cardiovascular/circulation.** Can interfere with clitoral engorgement needed for sexual response
- **Hyperlipidemia.** Elevated lipid levels can interfere with the blood flow to the pelvic area
- **Hyperglycemia.** Affects blood vessel integrity, mood changes, fatigue, headaches, and so forth

Janis recommends several basic treatments for increased pleasure that include: improved blood glucose control, following a Mediterranean diet, using a water-based lubricant estrogen therapy (e.g., cream, gel, tablet), changing depression meds if they are not working, using self-stimulation, and performing kegel exercises. Some sexual issues for women can include: an inability to achieve orgasm, decreased lubrication, pain/discomfort during intercourse, reduced libido, and lowered self-esteem (weight gain, injection/infusion set marks, etc.). Janis recommends some emotional treatments for increasing pleasure which include: making sure you are getting enough rest, participating in consistent physical activity, and using a reliable form of contraception. She also says that some people will have to change their expectations about pleasure, especially if they are unable to perform the way they did in the past. For example, they may have to expand their definition of pleasure to include actions other than intercourse. Or they may have to learn to appreciate smaller moments of pleasure such as long walks, holding hands, and so forth. Finally, Janis says it's important to remember that a good sex life requires more than a pill. Open communication is important to every relationship and remember that being positive and encouraging will go a long way.

Contraceptives

Women with diabetes need to educate themselves about contraceptives. The Centers for Disease Control and Prevention's (CDC) *Diabetes and Women's Health Across the Life Stages* reported:

> *Because intrauterine devices (IUDs) have been associated with an increased risk for pelvic infection, use among women with diabetes has previously been limited. However, several controlled studies using newer IUDs have shown them to be safe and effective in reproductive-aged women with diabetes. Low-dose combination oral contraceptives can also be used for contraception by women with diabetes. However, selection of the proper progestin and estrogen dosages for diabetic women to minimize potential adverse effects on glucose, lipid, and blood pressure should be considered.*

Janis recommends the following tips on birth control:

- Low-dose birth control pills
- Progesterone and high estrogen doses may alter glucose level
- IUD: increases chance of infections
- Diaphragm: may increase yeast infections
- Norplant or Depo-Provera: may affect glucose levels

Before she was ready for children, Annie Berger used the Nuvo Ring:

> *I thought this was a great option for diabetics because you put it in once every 4 weeks, but you don't have to worry about it every day—we have enough to worry about! I never noticed any impact it had on my blood sugar or any other side effects at all.*

Rachel Garlinghouse said that her sex drive increased and she lost 5 pounds when she stopped using the pill and many other women used condoms as their primary method of birth control.

Sex (Sometimes) Leads to Marriage

We all know that living with diabetes is stressful and many of us know that being married and maintaining a good relationship with our spouse is a great source of support. I will never forget the first time I got low with my husband. We were set up on a blind date by my mother and had been dating for a few weeks. He lived in Atlanta and would drive to Charleston almost every weekend so we could be together. One night, while we were standing in the kitchen, I felt my blood sugar started to drop. I'd told him about diabetes and had even explained to him how much it stressed me out when I would get low and my mom would start to act all crazy. I knew that it made her nervous to see my blood sugar drop, but I always felt like she overreacted, which then made me more defensive and irritable, and the entire event became bigger than it needed to be. He must have been paying attention because when I got low with him that first time, I remember he poured a glass of orange juice, set the glass next to me, and wandered away. I picked up the juice, drank it, and was fine within moments. I was so grateful for his calm approach, which helped me remain calm and not feel like I'd screwed up somehow. Eleven years later, he is still like that when I get low, calm and supportive, and that's exactly what I need.

Dr. Paula M. Trief, in an article that she wrote for Diabetes Self-Management's Web site, *Diabetes and Your Marriage: Making Things Work*, she says:

> *The quality of your relationship with your intimate partner can affect your general health and your diabetes control. Studies that have looked at the effect of marital stress on health have shown that your immune system, heart, and blood glucose control can all be negatively affected if you have a high degree of conflict and stress in your interactions with your partner. Your partner's involvement in your daily diabetes care can also make a lot of difference. It can make a positive*

> *difference if, for example, your partner prepares nutri-*
> *tious meals, keeps track of your medicines for you, or*
> *exercises with you.*[2]

Having diabetes can put a unique strain on a marriage, but it can also bring you closer if you learn to work together. Dr. Trief suggests:

- **Get educated.** This helps if both partners know what diabetes is, what must be done to manage it, and what to expect in the future.
- **Communicate.** Talk about what you both need from each other. Talk about what is helping and not helping. Try not to be critical of each other but to approach this conversation with an open, nondefensive attitude.
- **Listen.** Ask your partner how he feels about the changes you are mak-ing, and then listen to his response. Don't interrupt, don't argue, don't try to convince him that he's wrong; just listen, not just to his words, but also to the feelings that are being shared.
- **Set shared goals.** Set goals for your diabetes management, like walk-ing together after dinner, and talk about how to achieve them. In addi-tion, set goals for your relationship, like improving your communication, and talk about how to achieve that like setting time to talk.
- **Make room for negative emotions.** Although it helps to be positive, recognizing negative emotions is part of the coping process. By accept-ing and experiencing these emotions, you can come to terms with the emotional impact of diabetes. And by sharing these feelings with your partner, you will decrease the conflict and build intimacy in your relationship.
- **Get support from others.** Even though your partner may be your main source of support, allow yourself to turn to other family mem-bers and friends too.
- **Commit to nurturing the relationship.** If your relationship is in trouble, admit it, talk about it, and recommit yourself to nurturing the relationship.

Dr. Trief is working on another study of couples, where one spouse has type 2 diabetes, to examine ways on how to improve long-term behavior modification. She says that people with diabetes are more likely to stick to a healthy lifestyle when their partner is supportive. She says that because diabetes is a self-care disease, there often can be a lot of blame and guilt. She says the partner of someone with diabetes can feel angry if his or her loved one is not taking care of himself or herself and that they will need the communication skills to get past these issues. "The couple needs to work as a team to support one another," she says. "It's also important for the patient to recognize the effect on their partner."

Stella Biggs has been married for 10 years and says that she is blessed to have a husband who is actively involved in her diabetes management:

> *Of course, diabetes adds stressors to our relationship. We have a wonderful relationship and two great children. The only thing that comes in the way is my health. My husband told me he married me to spend the rest of his life with me and he still intends on doing that, but if my health gets in the way (by actively not taking care of myself, not by the disease and its everyday problems), it will be detrimental to our relationship. Diabetes affects everyone in our family: my husband, our two little girls, and me. I will be the one to ruin our relationship if I choose not to take care of myself. How can I help my family if I cannot help myself? (Reminds me of the air mask on the plane when your children are sitting with you.)*

Dr. William Polonsky of the Behavioral Diabetes Institute coined the term, "the diabetes police"[3] to refer to spouses who act more like a parent than a partner, asking if you've checked your blood sugar, what the numbers are, and should you really be eating that?

COMMUNICATION DYNAMICS

Ann Albright, PhD, RD, Director of the Division of Diabetes Translation at the Centers for Disease Control and Prevention, has type 1 diabetes. She says developing a philosophy about diabetes is key to long-term management. Dr. Albright's husband, who passed away 10 years ago, "always had his radar up" about her diabetes and "was incredibly supportive. He was able to find that wonderful balance of being aware and helpful without being overbearing."

She says this kind of relationship and family support help shape your philosophy of living with diabetes.

Developing diabetes later in life may require significant adjustments for a woman and her partner, especially for those in a new relationship. "Hopefully you're going to talk about your diabetes fairly soon. That decision depends on how you feel about your diabetes, how confident you are, how you express your frustration with your diabetes. All of those things are going to impact lots of parts of your intimate relationship, not just the sexual part. That's why having a much deeper relationship allows you to navigate through those issues with a lot less anxiety and frustration."

Rachel Garlinghouse says that diabetes brought her closer to her husband:

> *You know when you get married and vow to be together in sickness and in health? Well, we got the sickness part! We survived a difficult time. Diabetes will always be our "sickness," but it hasn't been all bad. We eat healthier now, exercise more, and chose to adopt two beautiful baby girls to avoid pregnancy. We are blessed.*

Lesley Hoffman Goldenberg says that she has a monthly diabetes *freak-out*:

> *I will just get to the point once in a while where the emotional burden of diabetes is too much for me to handle, and I feel so trapped. I think about how I will have it forever, and I can't get rid of it, and it makes me feel like I want to jump out of my skin. I think about my poor stomach and hip area that has endured multiple pump sites and how it hurts and how much it sucks. And I cry and punch my pillow and work through it, and then, I'm totally fine. I think that, sometimes, it makes Matt (my husband) sad and stresses him out because he wishes he could help me and make it go away. It doesn't put a strain on our relationship, but it just makes us both very, very sad.*

Stella Biggs had a boyfriend after college who was a registered dietician and worked in nursing homes. She says;

> *He saw a lot of older people die from diabetes complications. We were pretty serious and thinking about marriage,*

but he said he couldn't handle knowing that I was going to die from diabetes and that he would have to take care of me for the rest of my life (I hadn't gotten on the pump yet), and so, we broke up. That was really tough. So, my next serious boyfriend, who I am married to, didn't know as much about diabetes. He did a lot of research when we started getting serious and decided he could handle any complications. Actually, diabetes helped him make the decision to marry me because he knew I could not wait forever to have children, and we are happily married with 2 children now.

Diabetes has definitely complicated things, especially my severe lows while pregnant. But my husband is both supportive and the diabetes police (when I get lows, he has to yell at me to drink orange juice, etc.). He doesn't like doing that, especially around others who are unaware, and think that he is being bossy to me. I let him have his way on that, because it makes him feel like he is helping me. He likes to be active, but not a tyrant. It is a nice fit, and it works for us most of the time. I am extremely lucky to have a supportive husband who understands how hard this is on all of us and loves me just the same.

Dr. Trief says that there is another side to this story. "I also work with cancer patients and have seen that coping with something difficult can bring a couple closer together."

Rachel Garlinghouse says that initially, her husband attended appointments with her:

But I quickly became my own advocate and attended appointments alone. I wanted to be the first one to process my lab results, particularly my A1c. My husband has checked my sugar before when I'm too low to get out of bed, and he's, on occasion, had to help me treat a low because I would pass out if I attempted to get up and get a sugar source myself. My husband is very good about giving me my space. He never says, "Should you eat that?" or "What's your sugar?" He doesn't peek over my shoulder to check my meter. He waits for me to be ready to share information with him. We have a good sense of humor about diabetes. I joke that when I die and meet Jesus, He'll have a dessert buffet waiting for me. I'm blessed to have such a patient, understanding, and loving man in my life.

Lesley Hoffman Goldenberg says that her husband is as involved as he needs to be:

He sits with me when I change my site and wakes me up when he goes to bed (about 2 hours after me) so I can check my sugar, just in case. He also is very encouraging and knowledgeable about various diabetes terms. I also send him blog postings all the time of things that are interesting or that I want him to read. He's very curious and gets it, as well as anyone can who doesn't have diabetes. He doesn't come to doctor's appointments, but I don't ask him to nor do I need him to, at this point.

Taking the Next Step: Talking About Having Children

Taking the next step in a relationship often means talking about having children. This conversation can be more stressful or more emotionally complex for women with diabetes.

Lori Dubrow says that she and her husband talk about having children sometimes:

We are both on the fence and that is not because I have diabetes. I have never really been the kind of person who wanted to have a biological child. I have a real hard time with pregnancy. We have talked about alternate ways such as adoption or surrogacy and haven't really come to any real conclusion. I am 31 now and my window is closing. Not that rapidly but I don't want to put my body or any baby in further danger if we do decide to get pregnant by waiting too long. We are not ready at this point in time; that is one thing that we know for sure.

Lesley Hoffman Goldenberg thinks about having children many times during the day, every day:

> *However, I don't feel like I'm quite ready, and I'm worried my body can't handle it. Matt is ready to have kids and wants to start trying soon (keep in mind we got married 2 months ago!). He keeps telling me I can handle it and we will work on my A1c together. I keep reminding him that diabetes aside, there are lots of other issues with having kids—financial, space-wise, and so forth. Oh, and that whole we live in Manhattan and private schools cost $50,000 per year thing, which makes me want to move to rural Nebraska.*

AUTHENTIC ADVICE

- Rachel Garlinghouse says:
  I think when you find "the one," and that person is right for you, you will find that communication with that person regarding your diabetes will come naturally. I know it's cliché, but my husband is my best friend. I can tell him anything. Now, that doesn't mean I dump the diabetes burden on him all the time. I've learned that sometimes I can carry an issue with me and handle it on my own, but sometimes, I need help or simply need to vent.

- Stella Biggs says:
  I think if I were young and dating right now, after being on the pump for so long and knowing how to take care of myself, I would have talked about my diabetes sooner than later. Diabetes is a part of everything I do now, but I did not always see it that way. I am reminded at least 10 times a day, now, that I am diabetic, and I don't think that would be something I could hide in the dating life with the alarms, bells and whistles constantly going off. Also, because of the internet and blogs, it's much easier to talk about, as I only

had a couple of old people in my diabetes support groups before. Times have changed, and I am sure I would have changed with them if I were still dating.

■ Jennifer Ahn says:

Be open and honest from the start. If they have problems or think you are damaged goods from the diabetes, move on.

For some women, living with diabetes can add a certain weight to a relationship and can test the seriousness of someone's ability to commit. For others, diabetes may not change a thing. Dr. Albright says formulating a philosophy of living with diabetes will help us through the good and bad and will help us develop and maintain relationships that are supportive without being "overprotective." Having confidence in our physical selves and accepting ourselves as healthy, sexy women will allow others to see us that way too.

7   Working Girl: Diabetes at Work and School

Years ago, before I had children, I was a busy working girl as a department store manager at Saks Fifth Avenue. I was drawn to the job because of the glamour and the expensive clothes and ended up working in retail for almost 10 years. After several years with Saks Fifth Avenue, I started to get restless and wanted to have more money. Saks wasn't offering a high enough salary, so I quit and went to work for Banana Republic. Working as a department store manager at Saks, I was on my feet for most of the day, carrying boxes and stacks of clothes or moving display equipment. I liked the physical part of the work, but I also liked that at Saks, I could retreat to my dark office in the storage room and test my blood sugar or have a snack when I was low. Whereas at Banana Republic, I quickly discovered that I was expected to always be "on the floor."

On a Sunday morning, during my training period at Banana Republic, I met with my new coworkers to redesign the layout of the store for the winter collection. Lifting, moving, folding, and climbing on ladders, I quickly started to get low. I wanted to prove myself in front of this new crew and so I kept quiet, figuring we'd stop for a break shortly. However, we never stopped for a break, and I began to stumble around the store. I hadn't told anyone that I had diabetes. I remember one of the managers attempted to give me directions; I began mumbling, unable to make any sense. He was looking at me funnily and in my head, I was telling myself to "Go get sugar!" My vision started to flash and I felt like I was falling, but something prevented me from asking for help or from helping myself. Finally, I stumbled away, pretending I had to go to the bathroom. Then, I searched through my purse for some sugar, which I ate in private, feeling ashamed and stupid.

Looking back, I wonder how many times I've made situations much worse than they needed to be because of my pride or my shame about diabetes. I realize now that it would have not been a big deal that day to be upfront about needing certain accommodations, but I was unable to ask for help or reveal myself as being needy; because to me, being needy was a horrible sign of weakness.

TELLING COWORKERS

According to the Americans with Disabilities Act, you don't have to tell your coworkers about your condition; however, it's a good idea to let someone close to you know about it in case of an emergency.

Rosalind Joffee, the president of cicoach.com (an online resource for professionals with chronic illness) and the author of *Keep Working Girlfriend*, says that telling people at work should be done on a "need-to-know" basis. "Only disclose if you feel that diabetes is having an impact on your performance, otherwise you are opening up a can or worms." However, if you do decide to tell, don't assume that simply saying, "I have diabetes" is all you need to say. Rosalind advises that you need to be prepared to explain how your condition might affect your work life—*and have answers about how you're going to handle that.*[1]

ROSALIND'S TIPS

- Consider what you want to gain from the conversation.
- Figure out what you need to say.
- Be clear about the intended outcome. "What do you want to walk away with?" During the meeting, think about the biases against illness and ask yourself if you need to name the disease? Could this backfire?
- (What you say) Think about how your illness affects you. Focus on your ideas for improvement and in what you need, so you can work to your best ability. Actively look for input in a concrete way.
- (How you say it) In a matter of fact, straightforward, and knowledgeable tone, not throwing this on the boss's plate. Your language should be simple to understand.

MANAGING SUGARS AT WORK

Rachel Garlinghouse is a freelance writer and a part-time composition teacher at a university. She says:

> *My teaching job is fairly active—I'm moving around the classroom and heading up and down three flights of stairs (from my classroom to my office). However, I spend long hours grading stacks of essays. Freelance writing is a sedentary job. I freelance from home, so managing my sugars is no issue. At work, however, I never want to get low while teaching, so I usually check my blood sugar before teaching and sometimes during. My students are aware that I have diabetes, and I tell them I will sometimes eat during class. It's never been an issue.*

Lesley Hoffman Goldenberg is an education director at a conservative synagogue in midtown Manhattan. She says:

> *I am the principal of the religious (Hebrew) school, and I oversee adult education programming, family programs, and other holiday children's events. On days when there is no school, I basically have a desk job. On days when there is school or there are other events, I barely sit down and am running around like a crazy woman. Because I workout every morning, my sugars are very consistent during the day. I sometimes get low in the afternoon, right around when Hebrew school starts. It's like my body knows I'm about to get really busy so it plays a trick on me! I have a very low basal rate in the afternoon but I still get low sometimes. I try to have a banana or granola bar to help with the low.*

Testing on the Job

It is often difficult to find a place at work where we can check our sugars without drawing attention to ourselves and inviting questions.

Katie says:

> *I work in a doctor's office, so everyone I work with knows and are just great about it! In high school, I worked at a grocery store and let most of my coworkers know as well as supervisors—I was not looked at as "fragile" or treated differently because of it (except for the fact that they knew [how] to keep the cookies away from me!). All in all, I felt it was important for my coworkers to know in case of an emergency. It's also a great way to educate people about diabetes. The more comfortable I am telling people, the more they feel comfortable asking me questions, learning about the disease. And about the lady who doesn't like blood, well just tell her you're about to test and to look away!*

Rachel Garlinghouse says:

> *Everyone knows I have diabetes, because I was diagnosed in the middle of a semester and I looked very ill (underweight, exhausted). I have no issue with people knowing I have diabetes, mostly because I think it's a way to connect with other diabetics, and from a safety perspective, people need to know the name of your disease in case there were to be a medical emergency. I have two fantastic jobs, both of which I'm passionate about and believe in. I am at the university about 10 hours a week; however, I do much of my work (prepping, grading, answering student e-mails) from home. As far as my freelance job, I am my own boss. I can take on as much or as little work as I want. I am blessed to have a husband who is an excellent financial provider for our family (including the necessary excellent health insurance), so I do not feel pressure to bring in a certain dollar amount.*

Claire Blum is a certified diabetes educator who usually tells coworkers about her diabetes. She believes that it helps people to understand her better and is an opportunity to educate others about diabetes:

> *And, when my blood sugar is low I tend to get silly and am more laid back. I want people to know what to*

expect, without panicking or driving me crazy trying to help. There are times, however, when I do not tell . . . when I don't believe a person needs to know that much about me, or when telling distracts from the business at hand.

Lesley Hoffman Goldenberg doesn't usually tell people about her diabetes unless it comes up and is extremely relevant to the conversation:

If we're talking about medical benefits, I'll share that I'm diabetic. If someone's child was diagnosed with diabetes, I'll share that I have it. But I have been the director for 6 years and there are still several parents and lots of teachers who have no idea. I don't keep it a secret, but I certainly don't publicize it. These people are entrusting their children's life and education to me for several hours per week. Telling them I have diabetes almost always gets translated as uncontrolled diabetes and people get scared. It's easier to share this information when it's extremely relevant.

INSURANCE, THE BIG BAD WOLF

Diabetes is considered a *preexisting condition* and, until recently, that meant many insurance companies could deny health benefits to people with diabetes. I had no idea how much it costs to treat diabetes until I graduated from college and was no longer on my parent's health insurance. It was a rude awakening. Most of the jobs I could find as a recent graduate, with a Bachelor of Arts in Art History, were part time and offered low salary and no insurance benefits. After spending some time on COBRA, I eventually ended up in a retail job that was not personally inspiring but had good benefits. I remember feeling trapped in that job, because even though I was ready to leave and find something more fulfilling, I couldn't quit and risk being labeled as *preexisting* and not getting picked up again. Even with health insurance coverage through work, the cost of diabetes care is still high, which can increase stress. The U.S. Department of Health and Human Services (USDHHS) announced the establishment of a new Pre-existing Condition Insurance Plan (PCIP) that will offer coverage to uninsured Americans who have been unable to obtain health coverage because of a preexisting health condition.

The government has been working to provide health care for all Americans, and in 2014, insurers will be banned from discriminating against adults with preexisting conditions. Good health care coverage still has a long way to go for underinsured and low-income people with diabetes.

Annie Berger says, "Health benefits are always a factor when considering a job. I remember starting my first job out of college more quickly than I would have like, because I couldn't let my insurance lapse."

BALANCING WORK, LIFE, AND DIABETES

Managing our personal and working lives is always a challenge. Throw diabetes into the mix, and suddenly, there are more decisions to think about each day. Sometimes, I feel like I'm spinning through the house and can almost feel the silky cape flapping behind me as I race from the laundry to the dishes, homework, papers, grades, and crying baby. Suddenly, I realized that I tested my blood sugar 15 minutes ago and "oops!" I forgot to look at the results. Or, I realize I gave my bolus or injection and, in the middle of the craziness of this life, I forgot to eat. My job for the last 10 years has been a stay-at-home/work-from-home mom, which meant I was at home and could eat when I wanted (as long as there was no screaming child). Now, as I am venturing back into the working world, I find myself having to come up with more creative ways to stay on some sort of schedule. This creativity has included eating a ZonePerfect bar for lunch in the 10 minutes of free time that I have between the classes I teach. This is not the best approach and there are days that I ended up on the high side, but it works for now. I've learned that balance is a goal, not always a guarantee.

Lesley Hoffman Goldenberg works full time. She says:

I have Friday off but I often have to run programming or teach on the weekends. On the days where there's religious school, I'm often at work from around 10 am until, sometimes, 8 or 9 pm. I try to bring a healthy dinner or run out and get a salad in the middle of it all. But, I end up eating at work and synagogue food is so unhealthy! They always have bagels, fattening tuna or egg salad, and/or pizza. I can actually handle and count pizza pretty well, but it's not filling. So, the eating part and working late is definitely a challenge. The great part about my job is that I run my own show. I certainly have bosses, but I am very autonomous and can get my work done as I please. If I need to chat with a doctor during the day, log my blood sugars, or leave for an appointment, no one bothers me about it or even necessarily knows. It's wonderful and I am very grateful for this position.

My advice is to always place diabetes high on the priority list, either as the first item or as the second one. Don't let it slide down. It's hard and it can be challenging depending on what kind of work you do, but it's imperative and as important as work or family. Otherwise, work and family won't matter, and diabetes will take over your life. Put diabetes on the front burner so, eventually, you can put it on the back burner. It will never take care of itself but it can be so well controlled, that it will seem "easier."

Emily Wefelmeyer teaches high school math. Her first class is at 7 AM. She says:

I am not a morning person to begin with, so my mornings are pure chaos. The biggest challenge for me is when I have my infusion set come out as I am in the shower (only happens on the days that I hit snooze 3 too many times!) and have to replace it, get dressed, grab breakfast and lunch and still be [able] to [arrive at] work on time (we have to be there 5 minutes before the kids, so there is no extra room).

Luckily for me, I am in a section of the building where we all cover for each other, and the group of ladies that I'm with is fabulous. They have covered my classes if I don't make it in because I need to change sets, they have covered for 3 minutes when I had to go back on shots, and they have covered for the last 5 minutes of the day so that I can make a doctor's appointment on time. I would not know what to do without them.

Jennifer Ahn is a maternal–fetal medicine specialist dealing with high-risk pregnancies. She says:

> *Some days, I have to be at work by 7 AM, other days at 8 AM.*
> *I usually work until 4:30 or 5 PM, depending on my day. I*
> *am on call two times a month, which requires me to stay*
> *overnight at the hospital. I try to exercise either in the AM*
> *(6-7) or in the evening after work. It has been a little more*
> *challenging of late as I recently moved in with my fiancé . . .*
> *so work/life and health balance are a little off sometimes,*
> *especially because my commute is now a lot longer. But,*
> *he understands that work and exercise are important to*
> *me. So, I tend to wake up around 4 to 4:30 AM to get things*
> *done and get my workout in. Not a problem as I am an*
> *early bird.*

Claire Blum's work schedule can be very stressful. She says:

> *My schedule is generally irregular and unpredictable, but*
> *I come prepared for whatever happens, and test, eat, bolus,*
> *treat lows, and care for my diabetes as an integrated part*
> *of my life. I just do it and keep going. Most of the time*
> *people are totally unaware of what I am doing. I remember*
> *going out to eat with a group of health care professionals,*
> *and sitting next to a diabetes educator who was entirely*
> *amazed that I had checked my [blood glucose] BG and*
> *given a bolus, without her notice . . . all the while carrying*
> *on a conversation.*

Managing Work-Related Stress

Rachel Garlinghouse feels confident and comfortable in her job, but admits that diabetes never ceases to surprise her:

> *Though I don't have a lot of work stress, diabetes is a*
> *full-time job in itself. Some days, especially after a series of*
> *bad highs and lows, it's very hard for me to go to work.*
> *But I feel a sense of responsibility to go, even if I'm not*
> *feeling well, because I'm only there 2 days a week. I have,*

*on occasion, called in sick, but most times I just trudge
through the day. I've found that lying around at home can
sometimes make me feel worse, because then I focus on
the negative effects of my disease. Feeling responsible for
the writing educations of my students pushes me to get
through bad days.*

Eating at Work

An important part of successfully managing our health is eating well at
work. That means stopping to eat when you are in the middle of a proj-
ect or bringing in a healthy lunch instead of eating from the vending
machine.

Claire Blum says that in the past, she was prone to allow work to take
precedence over eating:

*I could not be bothered to take the time to eat or prepare
healthy meals. My meals often consisted of prepackaged food
that kept my blood sugar from dropping, but provided little
nutrition. As a result of my poor nutritional intake, and
other medical challenges, my health declined a great deal.
Since then, I have learned to pay attention to my body's
signals and find that preparing and carrying food that is
healthy for my body not only helps me feel better . . . it also
helps me achieve the things I most want to do!*

AUTHENTIC ADVICE

- Lesley Hoffman Goldenberg says:
  *My advice is to always place diabetes high on the priority
  list—either as the first item or as the second one. Don't let it slide
  down. It's hard and it can be challenging depending on what
  kind of work you do, but it's imperative; it's as important as work
  or family. Otherwise, work and family won't matter and diabetes will take over your life. Put diabetes on the front burner so*

eventually, you can put it on the back burner. It will never take care of itself but it can be so well controlled that it will seem "easier."

■ Claire Blum says:

Honor and care for your body . . . Your dreams depend on it!

■ Rachel Garlinghouse says:

I'm a strong believer in this: Women, especially those with a chronic illness, must put themselves first. If you don't take care of yourself, how will you take care of others in the ways they need and desire? My husband, my daughter, my parents, my students, my friends—they deserve the very best from me! So I take my disease seriously. I say "no" often, because I take working out, cooking healthy meals, and making time to relax very seriously. Once a woman decides she is worthy of a healthy mind, body, and spirit and she takes steps to cultivate healthy wholeness, she will become the best partner, mother, employee, friend, [and] daughter that she can be.

I love my work; I love interviewing people for my freelance assignments and teaching students how to write the five-paragraph essay. People say, "Do what you love to do and happiness or money will follow," and I believe that to be true. Living with diabetes is often compared to a full-time job or a third (or fourth!) child. However, it doesn't have to be our only job or our only child. We need to figure out how to make room for more than managing our illness. Finding fulfillment with the work we are passionate about makes for a well-balanced life, and the more balanced we are, the better we feel.

8   Travel

I spent a semester in Italy during my junior year of college. I kept a journal while I was living in Florence, and the first entry from that semester is dated January 9, 1991. I wrote:

> *The first sounds I heard as I came to in the hospital were foreign. Rapid, tight Italian words that bounced above my head between bodies dressed in white. I thought I was having a nightmare. The room was stark white with bright lights, and the equipment was bulky, boxy, and outdated. The equipment they used to test my blood sugar was ancient-large and heavy with wires. There were other patients in the room, older patients who were staring and talking at me, and I couldn't understand any of them. I was soaked with sweat, bloody, and they were feeding me straight sugar. Then a woman came in from the college and she started to explain what happened and everything slowly came back to me.*

On my first morning in Florence, my new friends and I went back to bed after breakfast because we were still adjusting to the time change. Italian breakfasts of bread, jam, and coffee are lower in carbs than my normal breakfast of cereal and milk, and my whole schedule was thrown off. I was sharing a room at a hotel with some other students during that first week until we were placed with our Italian families. One of the students had a friend back home who had diabetes and recognized the signs of low blood sugar in me. The rest of the girls woke up at 10 AM to get ready for the day, but were unable to wake me. They told me later that I was sweaty and moaning in bed, and they called one of the teachers who called an ambulance. I was carried out of the hotel on a stretcher past all the other students and taken by ambulance to the local hospital.

Days later, settling into the room I shared with another American student in our Italian family's home. I sat on my small bed and allowed myself to remember that fateful morning. I didn't want to think about it. I wanted to press it to the depths of my mind, but the images kept surfacing, and so, I sat down to remember everything and wrote it in my journal.

Regaining consciousness was terrifying. I heard a foreign language spoken too quickly for me to understand, as I was pulled from the depths of the murky, heavy water of unconsciousness. No, no, don't let this happen! No, not again! I wanted to return to the dark, quiet place. I didn't want to wake up because waking up meant that it was real.

I talked to my mom on the phone that night, and we agreed that I would be fine. We concluded that my low blood sugar had occurred because of the different foods I ate and the time change, and decided that I would continue with the program. Looking back, I know that I wanted my mom to insist that I come home. I remember walking away from the phone after our conversation and feeling shocked that she hadn't even asked if I wanted to come home. A part of me did want to go home—the part of me that had been terrified by the whole experience in the Italian hospital and was scared of the seemingly uncontrollable powers within my body. But I didn't want to admit I was scared, so I stayed.

A week or two later, my early renaissance class took a field trip on January 20—my birthday—to visit Santa Croce, the principal Franciscan church in Florence and also the burial place of Michelangelo. Inside the church are the frescoes painted by Giotto. That afternoon, I stood in a large circle with my classmates and listened to our teacher, explaining the history of the church and the art; then, I began to stumble. I swayed around, bumping to the other students who were standing next to me. I saw my leather backpack at my feet; I'd bought it for myself as an early birthday present at the market in the middle of the city. It was beautiful soft brown leather, and inside the front pocket were lemon and strawberry Italian candies. I stared at my backpack, it held something I needed, but I couldn't move. A girl standing next to me asked me if I wanted to get some air. I nodded and reached down and grabbed my backpack. I stumbled away from the crowd and sat down in the middle of the cathedral. I began to dig through my backpack, searching for a candy, but couldn't really see any. So, I got up again and tried to go outside. Katie, a girl from our group, came over to ask if I was okay.

"I just need some air," I managed to say. The words felt thick like honey on my tongue. I stumbled out of the darkened church into the sunlight. The buzzing noises of the mopeds on the narrow streets startled me, and I stumbled backward, coming to rest with my back against the church walls. My vision was flashing as I leaned against the side of the church, melting into the cold stones. The same girl (Katie) came out after me, then there were two guys holding onto me, and then, we rode a cab. The students took me back to school and carried me into the nurse's office, and then called for an ambulance. This time, I was given an intravenous (IV) of sugar at the school and my strength quickly came back. My roommate was there and she sat with me until I felt better. After I stopped shaking, she walked with me out of the nurse's office through the school, and out onto the street to wait for the bus home.

As I wrote the story in my journal, I felt sorry for myself. I was ashamed, embarrassed, depressed, and homesick. I was alone and hated my disease. Looking back now, I'm glad that my parents didn't insist I come home because living in Italy was one of the greatest experiences of my life. It was also one of my greatest challenges in life because I realized that I had to depend on myself and I did. I didn't have a bad low for the rest of the semester, instead, I figured out how to have an unforgettable experience.

AIR TRAVEL AND DIABETES

I remember a weekend trip to New York City for a wedding; and the morning we were supposed to fly home, a snowstorm hit and our flight was canceled. I was at the very end of my bottle of insulin and had to find a pharmacy to buy another bottle. I didn't have a prescription and I think it was a Sunday, so I was unable to call my doctor's office at home, so I had to pay full price for the insulin. I was frustrated at myself, at the weather, the pharmacy, and the fact that I had diabetes at all. It was the end of a great weekend and a rude reminder of my responsibilities. Looking back, I wish I could say that I've learned my lesson since that day,

TIPS ON AIR TRAVEL

- See your doctor before you go. Get a letter describing your diabetes management and a copy of your prescriptions.
- Whenever possible, bring prescription labels for medication and medical devices (Although not required by TSA, making them available will make the security process go more quickly).
- Pack medications in a separate clear bag and place in your carry-on luggage.
- Keep a quick-acting source of glucose to treat low blood glucose (glucose tabs), as well as an easy-to-carry snack such as a nutrition bar.
- Carry or wear medical identification (a cute diabetes bracelet) and carry contact information for your physician.
- Pack extra supplies, at least twice as much medication and supplies as you think you'll need.
- Keep supplies in a carry-on bag.
- Because prescription laws may be very different in other countries, write for a list of International Diabetes Federation groups (IDF, 1 rue Defaeqz, B-1000, Belgium) or visit http://www.idf.org. You may also want to get a list of English-speaking foreign doctors in case of an emergency. Contact the American Consulate, American Express, or local medical schools for a list of doctors. Insulin in foreign countries comes in different strengths. If you purchase insulin in a foreign country, be sure to use the right syringe for the strength. An incorrect syringe may cause you to take too much or too little insulin.

but I can count on both hands the times I've run into trouble while traveling, and have had to scramble to get my hands on test strips or a pump or insulin. I think I must have some sort of emotional stubbornness that kicks in when it comes to travel or an inability to plan appropriately for my trip, and I end up in a state of panic and short on supplies. One of the most frustrating parts of diabetes is that you never become an expert.

After 25 years of living with this disease, I still make mistakes. And even though I try not to beat myself up when I go for a run, forget to bring glucose tabs and get low, or go out of town for the weekend and run out of test strips, I feel like I have no one to blame but myself. So I'm gathering as much information as I can offer to my readers, but I'm also laying my own cards on the table and saying, I screw up all the time, don't expect perfection.

Lesley Hoffman Goldenberg's rule is to always pack double of what she'll need on her trip:

> *I always make up a scenario that I get stranded in whatever country I'm traveling to or that I have to change my site every day, since it's going to get ripped out every single day. Therefore, I always travel with double (which you see is based on no logic whatsoever). When traveling internationally, I always bring the phone numbers of their local MiniMed or pump supply companies, just in case. I always, always travel with a travel pump that MiniMed so graciously lets us borrow for about $50. It's the best and makes me feel so safe and secure!*

Linda Frick has been traveling for pleasure since the year 2000:

> *At first, I would wear my pump in my bra like I normally do, and the airport metal detector would never alarm. As the airport security got tighter over time at some airports, the battery in my pump would make the metal detector alarm, and it was at that point I started wearing it on my waistband as they will not let you move it once you are picked out of line for a pat down procedure. I do have issues with TSA staff touching my pump. I have had them wipe down my pump with their cloth for gunpowder testing and I believe they need more extensive training on touching the pump. I also have learned to never ever wear a long skirt as a woman going through the checkpoint. There is nothing more humiliating and frustrating than a TSA agent frisking your inner thighs while the whole world is watching!*

Kristin Makszin is currently living in Budapest, Hungary, working on her PhD in political science. She was diagnosed in 2003, at the age of 21, with type 1 diabetes; she is a frequent globe-trotter:

> *I have had many lows while traveling, but just treated them like I usually would. Always have something with you to treat your low. While traveling on a plane, make sure that it is in the seat pocket or under the seat so that you can access it even when you must keep your seat belt fastened.*

> *When I am traveling by plane by myself, I always order a diabetic meal. The food is not always low carb, but usually a bit fresher and healthier than the other meal (though sometimes a bit more bland too!). The main reason that I order it is then the flight attendant also knows that I have diabetes. If there was an emergency, that could be helpful!*

> *Most of my travels were while I was studying abroad. So I would make international trips at least once a year. I have also traveled a lot within Europe (by train, plane, or bus) while I have been studying there. The only inconvenience is always needing to carry more than enough supplies and food. By planning ahead, traveling with diabetes should be just like traveling without diabetes.*

> *Diabetes was never really a problem during my travels. I love traveling and I am so thankful that diabetes never prevented me from exploring the world!*

Crossing Time Zones

If you take insulin shots and will be crossing time zones, talk to your doctor or diabetes educator before your trip. Bring your flight schedule and information on time zone changes. Your doctor or educator can help you plan the timing of your injections while you travel.

Kristin Makszin says:

> *You should change the time on your pump. For example, I usually do a 6-hour time change, and during the flight, I change it back/forward 2 hours, three times. If the time*

change is more than 2 hours, then don't do it all at once!
This is particularly important if you have drastic differ-
ences in your basal levels throughout the day.

TIPS WHEN TRAVELING BETWEEN DIFFERENT TIME ZONES

- Remember, eastward travel means a shorter day. If you inject insulin, less may be needed. Westward travel means a longer day, so more insulin may be needed.
- To keep track of shots and meals through changing time zones, keep your watch on your home time zone until the morning after you arrive.
- If you inject insulin while in flight, frequent travelers suggest being careful not to inject air into the insulin bottle. In the pressurized cabin, pressure differences can cause the plunger to resist. This can make it hard to measure insulin accurately.
- Check your blood glucose while traveling as you would when you're at home.
- In addition, check your blood glucose level as soon as possible after landing. Jet lag can make it hard to tell if you have very low or very high blood glucose.

Lesley Hoffman Goldenberg says that when she travels within the United States, the time change doesn't usually affect her sugars:

I usually change my pump clock about 3 hours after I land
in a new location and am starting to do activities that are
different than what I would be doing at home. When I
travel internationally, I usually do the same thing actually.
I just carefully monitor my blood sugars and try not to get
the trip really going until I've been there at least a day.

Traveler's Insurance

Travel insurance is purchased to cover travel-related risks, including last-minute cancellations because of sickness, severe weather, or even terrorist attacks. Insurance also provides coverage for emergency/accident care, medical evacuations, travel delays and missed connections, lost/stolen baggage, and more. Travel medical insurance is purchased by travelers leaving their home country for a few days or up to a year and provides emergency medical treatment, medical evacuation coverage, and emergency assistance.

Travel medical policies are for travelers who are going overseas and need medical insurance. When you travel outside your home country, your health insurance from home might not cover you. If it does, the limits might be too low to cover the expenses, or it might not cover your medical evacuation costs. There are over 15 companies in the travel insurance business, and each one sells various plans. Some companies specialize in simple, easy-to-use policies for the everyday traveler. In general, the premium amount for a travel medical plan is based on the length of the trip, the age of the traveler, and the amount of coverage.

Kristin Makszin says that most travel health insurances don't cover diabetes, because it is considered a preexisting condition. She says, "Many insurance plans can be used outside of the United States for a certain number of days (mine used to be 90), but for longer than that, it might be difficult to find insurance coverage for diabetes."

Whenever Linda Frick travels outside of the United States, she always purchases travel insurance that includes medical and medical evacuation in the event that she needs to be transported back home:

Thankfully, I have never had to use this insurance. I also always travel with a family member or friend who knows my health needs and can respond appropriately. Several years ago, I was in Hong Kong with my father, and we were sightseeing with a group of travelers who seemed to have very long legs and speed-walked/ran everywhere. Now, I'm only 5 feet 3 inches with short little legs, so you can imagine how hard it was for me to keep up with them. Not knowing how much exercise I would be getting can be difficult, and sometimes, I have to do things by trial and error. Well, we walked so fast and so long that I had an abrupt hypoglycemic episode and my legs collapsed. Also, since I've been diabetic for so long (going on 50 years now) I have hypoglycemia unawareness and can't always tell when I'm going low. I grasped and hung on to the

*closest thing to me (which happened to be a light pole) and
waited for my group (including my father) to realize that I
was down. Of course, they immediately came to my rescue
once they looked back and wondered what had happened
to me and fed me candy. I did have candy on me but
because the incident happened so quickly, I did not have
time to respond. Of note, no one in the large city metropo-
lis came to my rescue other than those that knew me.
I could clearly see that many thought I was intoxicated.
I do wear a medic alert bracelet at all times.*

PACKING AND PLANNING

Ann Rosenquist Fee spent part of the winter and spring of 2010 in Port
Elizabeth, South Africa with her visiting-professor-husband and son. She
tells us:

*Port Elizabeth is a perfectly modern place with a drug
store called Clicks, open daily until 1700 inside the
Summerstrand Village mall across from Hobie beach on
the Indian Ocean.*

*Several times a week, in the warm clear wash of African
sun, I walked the 45-minute walk from our flat in a
graduate student village to the beachfront. Then, I walked
barefoot in the sand parallel with Beach Drive until it was
time to cross the street into Summerstrand Village.*

*I never had a long shopping list. Living in a less
consumer-oriented culture had reduced my shopping
libido. And I'd brought along most of what I really
needed for my 4-month stay, including the majority of
my diabetic supplies—syringes, test strips, long-acting
and short-acting insulin. But I'd counted on South Africa
to have glucose tablets available for purchase, possibly
in local flavors like litchi or guava.*

*About the time I lost my patience for the long hot walks,
the relatively limited selections and hours in drug and
grocery stores, the conspicuousness of my accent, and the*

subtle, constant racism of which I was implicitly guilty as a white person, I needed glucose. Not immediately, but I needed to replenish my supply of the tablets I'd brought from home.

The Clicks clerk just blinked and waved me to the pharmacy. The pharmacist walked me back over to where the clerk was, by the hard candy section. "You could buy sweets," one of them said. I don't remember which one. I just remember feeling enraged on behalf of South African diabetics forced to wait for some damn orange-chocolate thing to melt in their mouth, if they could afford to buy such a luxury in a country where the majority lived well below the poverty level. And I remember missing the tart, chalky taste of tablets that come in plastic tubs at American pharmacies where diabetes, like most other things, is cushioned by 24-hour access, wild variety, and the pretense that the customer is always right.

Rachel Garlinghouse says that some of the biggest challenges of traveling as a woman with diabetes are packing:

My "master packing list" (and yes, I created one so I wouldn't forget anything crucial) is lengthy. My purse is always large (no cute little designer bags for me!) to accommodate my diabetes supplies. Packing is the biggest challenge with traveling, because I really don't want to forget anything. Having diabetes means I am constantly aware of my body and what I do to it. When I eat, whether at home or when traveling, I do so with my diabetes and my overall health in mind. That doesn't mean I don't eat dessert, but it does mean that I don't pig out on appetizers, then a huge entree, and then a dessert. I carefully calculate and balance my meals. I exercise while on vacation, just like I do at home. Some people look at exercise as a chore, but really, it's a privilege. And I know if I choose not to workout, I am choosing to feel bad later. I was at the hotel gym on Thanksgiving morning this year. I was the only person in there, but I told myself that I was doing a good thing for my body—physically and emotionally.

Lesley Hoffman Goldenberg loves visiting new places and learning about new cultures and says that the key to a good time is planning:

> *I've been to Europe for 3 weeks with a close friend. I've been to Israel five times and to Italy, Switzerland, Poland, Czech Republic, Jordan, and Spain. I try very hard to prepare for each and every trip I take in terms of my diabetes. I read up on different cultures and try to educate myself so I know what kind of food to expect and how to roughly count it. I also travel with hundreds of glucose tablets, since I'm usually walking a lot and constantly on the go. I usually just give myself some time off while I travel so that I can fully enjoy myself and not let the big D drag me down.*

Linda Frick says that her first travel experience was in 2000, when she was invited to go to Italy with her neighbors:

> *It was after that wonderful trip that I knew that I had a traveler's bug to see the world. Since that trip, I've been to many other places—China, New Zealand, and Mexico City to name a few. The air travel time to China (as well as New Zealand) was quite lengthy (at 14 hours) and played havoc with my blood sugars. Sitting with very little exercise for that length of time, other than walking up and down the crowded plane aisle, did little to keep my blood glucose levels where they should be. My trip to China was wonderful! I walked on the Great Wall, saw the Forbidden City in Beijing, and sailed on the Li River to Guilin. I bolused my way through most of China and enjoyed their diverse array of foods and fruits without any major problems other than elevated glucose levels at times.*

EATING ABROAD

Kristin Makszin spent a year in rural Ukraine with her pump and says that her diet consisted of mostly bread and butter:

> *Protein was not very available unless you had your own chickens (maybe I should have gotten chickens). My blood*

sugars were not awesome that year, but I kept my A1c under 8 and it was definitely worth it, as it was an amazing year!

I took all my pump supplies, insulin, test strips with me. I did not see a doctor that year at all (I could have seen someone in the nearest city if there was an emergency). I adjust my own basal rates on the pump and took a couple of the A1c home tests with me to check on myself.

My doctor never discouraged me from going. She even gave me tips on adjusting basal rates before I left. I could get eggs in the village—thankfully, I love eggs and ate about 20 eggs per week. It was the village gossip to talk with the shopkeeper about my egg consumption!

AUTHENTIC ADVICE

- Rachel Garlinghouse says:
  I think succeeding with diabetes is all about planning, and traveling with the disease is no different. Create a master packing list that you can refer to before you travel, making sure to list individual supplies (test strips, syringes, etc.) so you do not forget anything. I make sure to put sandals in my bag so I can easily slip them on and wear them in the hotel (foot safety!). I pack tons of extra supplies, and I carry identification on me at all times. These small things add up to my peace of mind when I'm traveling.
- Lesley Hoffman Goldenberg says:
  As I've mentioned many, many times, you must always be prepared. Bring more than you need even if it means checking an extra bag. Send yourself extra supplies to the hotel or person's house where you're staying. Never check the medical supplies (in baggage check) and always have them with you. Just bring lots and lots and lots of extra supplies. Get your doctor to write a travel letter so you can flash that if there's a problem. And, always get that travel pump from MiniMed or from

whatever pump company you need. I have used it once but it made me feel a lot less nervous and more secure while traveling. Whenever I pack clothes or anything in general, I go through each day and what I need throughout my entire routine. I do that with diabetes too—I wake up and what do I do? I check my blood sugar. Okay, pack tons of testing strips and granola bars for the morning. I get a low blood sugar mid-morning, because I'm walking around a lot so what do I need? I need glucose tablets and a purse that can fit glucose tablets and extra goodies. Okay, pack that. I take my site out at night and it's red and infected so how do I treat that? I need to pack Neosporin and possibly, a prescription for an antibiotic to cure that. I find if you go through an entire routine, you'll remember everything you need. The key is to always be prepared, have a sense of humor, and be extremely patient.

■ Linda Frick says:

Learn to adjust and go off schedule. Traveling can be very non-routine and you must be flexible. You may not always be able to eat from the food groups associated with your diabetic diet—learn to adlib and enjoy!

My parents didn't ask me to leave Italy because of my low blood sugars. Even though I was hurt and confused, I realized that being there on my own taught me to ask for help. I did better than to survive the trip; I had an experience that went beyond my expectations. Moreover, I began to learn how to accept help from friends, teachers, and even strangers when it comes to my diabetes.

9   Pregnancy

Diabetes was low on my priority list until I started thinking about becoming a mother. This body that I'd used to propel me from one risk-taking adventure to the next (hiking in the Grand Canyon, running a marathon, and jumping out of a plane) now needed to be treated kindly. My doctor explained that the first weeks of pregnancy were the most important for a baby's development. He said my blood sugars needed to be in tight control to ward off birth defects and I was paralyzed with fear. I was not even pregnant yet, and there was so much at stake. *Birth defects*—two terrible words. I'd always acted like I was different from other people with diabetes and that the complications were not a concern of mine because I would be different; I would be fine. But birth defects? My diabetes had never physically affected anyone other than me.

My husband and I tried to get pregnant for a year. Each month was a disappointment, and I began to think I wasn't meant to be a mother, that maybe my body was defective in more ways than one. In the dark places of my heart, I feared that my body—this body that I injected, pricked, fed, and denied like a science experiment—might deny me this basic, fundamental female skill. Having been betrayed by my body at the edge of adolescence, I feared another internal malfunction. I was terrified that I would be excluded from the experience of motherhood.

So, I worked really hard to do everything correctly. I tested my sugars obsessively, ate balanced meals, cut out caffeine, and exercised. After 6 months of trying and failing to get pregnant, I began my first round of fertility drugs.

A few days before Christmas, I knew something was different with my body. Having diabetes demands a certain intimacy with my body; I'd learned at a young age to read my body signals like a foreign language. If I yawned in the middle of the morning, maybe my blood sugar was dropping; or if my jaw felt tight, my blood sugar was probably spiking. My breasts were sore and that was unfamiliar. I stood in the shower and pressed my hands against the sides of my breasts, one after the other; and they were sore, I was not imagining things. I was pregnant.

The thrill of pregnancy quickly transformed into the science of management. Labeled "high risk," the threat of birth defects floated, just beneath the surface of my pregnancy. I was closely monitored, measured, tested, weighed, poked, and prodded for 9 months by a team of doctors. I ate low-carb meals and snacks, even though what I really wanted was a thick slice of peanut butter toast. I tested my blood sugar so often that my fingertips were harder and more calloused than they'd ever been. Every time I got a "bad" reading (.180 mg/dl), I was plagued by guilt and imagined that the sugar was flowing like poison through my blood and into my baby. In the high-risk room of the local hospital, I held my breath every time I had an ultrasound, worrying about what I might see in those blurry images. I tried to read the face of the technician for clues, but her eyes were flat and unblinking.

I worked hard to avoid bad readings and low blood sugars. I worked hard to exercise, take my vitamins, and go to all my doctor appointments, but I also watched my friend at work who was due a few weeks before me and listened to her talk about taking long baths, sleeping late on the weekend, drinking milkshakes, and I burned with envy. It sounded so easy. I struggled to think positive thoughts, to visualize a healthy baby, and to treat my body less like a machine and more like a mother-to-be. On August 28, 2001, our son was born.

When I went back on Clomid to get pregnant with Miles, 2 years later, I wasn't as fearful. I understood that my body required additional medical assistance, like insulin and Clomid, to survive, to function, and to perform these normal biological tasks. I know the risks to a child born to a diabetic mother. Before the discovery of insulin in the 1920s, pregnancy in women with diabetes was a life-threatening experience. Even afterward, for years, women struggled to maintain healthy pregnancies. With the help of medical advances in managing care, the risks have decreased, but not disappeared.

I am now a 40-year-old type 1 diabetic mother to three healthy boys. My last pregnancy occurred without any fertility drugs and was in fact a surprise. Even though I was older, I felt stronger and wiser and less fearful about the whole experience. My children have been the motivation for me to get myself in good health and to remain in good health. My three pregnancies have felt like affirmations that this body—this damaged body—is in fact fertile and able in its own way.

FERTILITY ISSUES

Janis Roszler says that diabetes can affect a woman's fertility for various reasons:

- Reproductive period may be reduced
- Delayed menarche
- Premature menopause
- Decreased desire limits sexual activity around ovulation
- Metformin (in polycystic ovary syndrome [PCOS]) decreases the testosterone production, however, ovulation may return after a few months
- Glycemic control increases fertility rates

More and more women with diabetes are having children than ever before. The Centers for Disease Control and Prevention's (CDC) report, *Diabetes and Women's Health Across the Life Stages,* states that between 1980 and 1996, the prevalence among females younger than 45 years of age remained steady until 1989, then increased by 27 percent, from 7.3 per 1,000 in 1989 to 9.3 per 1,000 in 1996. An approximately 70 percent increase in diabetes prevalence among women aged 30–39 years of age has been noted between 1990 and 1998. . . . The rapid changes in these risk factors among reproductive-aged women suggest a population wide impact of social and environmental factors. Moreover, they also suggest that increasing numbers of women, especially nonwhite women, are now at risk for having pregnancies complicated by diabetes.

HISTORY OF DIABETIC PREGNANCIES

Dr. Priscilla White worked with Dr. Joslin at the famous Joslin Center in Massachusetts and was one of the leading researchers in diabetic pregnancies. Before the discovery of insulin in the 1920s, pregnancy in women with diabetes was a life-threatening experience. Even afterward, for years, women struggled to maintain a healthy pregnancy. Dr. White passed away in 1989, after working tirelessly to improve the lives of women and children with diabetes. She is quoted as saying, "Before insulin, coma was the end-result of the pregnant diabetic. No matter what course was adopted, the danger was imminent. Surgical intervention with general anesthesia would precipitate it. Fetal death, which occurred in 50 percent of the cases prior to insulin, was a source of coma. If the patient came successfully to term, labor accompanied by partial starvation and overexertion would bring it on."[1]

Dr. White undertook meticulous research into many aspects of diabetes and, in particular, into aspects aimed at improving the outcome of pregnancy for both the mother and the child. By the time of her retirement, the fetal survival rate for diabetic women in the Joslin Clinic had risen from 54–97 percent. She is known for her classification system of pregnant diabetic women and fetal survival rates in an attempt to correlate the severity of diabetes and health of the pregnancy.

With the help of medical advances in managing daily care, the risks have decreased, but have not disappeared.

Linda Frick has been a type 1 diabetic for 50 years and has lived through the improvements in prenatal care. The first time she got pregnant was in 1974, before there were home glucose monitors. She was taking one shot of insulin a day and did not monitor her blood sugars:

> *My denial had me convinced that I could have a normal pregnancy like "everybody" else. Sadly, my pregnancy ended when my baby died at 7 months in utero. I'm sure it was due to my lack of adequate control, and my poor choice of doctor who did not know much about controlling my disease during pregnancy. I had preeclampsia and liver problems along with very high blood pressure. I'm sure my life was at risk as well.*

> *My second pregnancy was by accident (IUD failure) in 1977. I had been so traumatized by the first pregnancy that I secluded myself from all others with children and did not want to set myself up for failure again. When I learned I was pregnant, I was excited and very, very scared. Back then, there were no Internet or mass informational resources. I often felt like I was the only pregnant diabetic in the world! I immediately set up an appointment with a doctor who would help me succeed. I was placed on a very strict diet, no salt, no caffeine, and [I] felt like I was starving myself to death but the payoff was going to be great! There was still no*

home blood glucose testing at that time, however, I went into the hospital every 1 to 2 weeks to have blood taken from my arm; I was on multiple daily injections by this time. I had diabetes for 16 years when my first child was born. I was hospitalized 3 weeks prior to my delivery time to ensure that I could be watched closely. Even while in the hospital and under their care, I developed preeclampsia and liver problems again. My daughter was born by cesarean section at approximately 37 weeks' gestation.

My denial of my chronic disease was immediately brought to the surface when I lost my first child. It's unfortunate that it sometimes takes a traumatic event to take control of your health.

THE *STEEL MAGNOLIAS* MYTH

I remember seeing the movie *Steel Magnolias* when I was a senior in high school and leaving the theater in tears. I knew that the movie was based on a true story about a young woman with diabetes who died from kidney failure. Seeing the movie was a powerful moment, because when I was diagnosed at 14 years old, the concept of motherhood was vague and distant. I still didn't imagine myself as anyone's mother as a senior in high school, but I had never imagined that I couldn't either. *Steel Magnolias* was a horror movie for thousands of young women with diabetes, setting fire to the fear that having children and becoming a mother would be a death sentence. It's been 20 years since the movie was released and even though advances in diabetes care and education has proven that women with diabetes can have healthy pregnancies and healthy babies, the myth and fear of *Steel Magnolias* remains strong.

Lori Dubrow says that she doesn't want a 22-pound baby:

I do have fears. I am afraid that I won't be able to keep it together during pregnancy and that my child will be sick as a result of me. I am also extremely afraid of having a child with diabetes. I don't know if that is a selfish thing on my part (not wanting the added responsibility of a child with diabetes) or if I would feel guilty that I gave this to my child.

Kristin Makszin says that the extra worries about pregnancy were one of the hardest challenges that came along with her diabetes diagnosis:

When I was diagnosed as a young adult (at age 21), I was not yet close to being ready to have children, but the issue weighed heavily on my mind and already caused me great stress and emotional turmoil. Once, after I was diagnosed, someone casually made a comment that their daughter couldn't get pregnant because of diabetes, I knew it was not true, but I still left the room in tears. Also, I know that every pregnant woman must be responsible for the health of their child, but the added responsibility of blood sugar maintenance meant that I waited longer to have children than I would have otherwise.

EDUCATION AND PREPREGNANCY PLANNING

In "Prevent Birth Defects: Don't Get Pregnant until Your Sugar Is Controlled," Linda von Wartburg wrote, "Over 70 percent of birth defects in babies of women with diabetes could be prevented by preconception care. If you take steps before pregnancy, your chance of having a healthy baby rises to that of the general population."[2] Sweet Success, a California Diabetes and Pregnancy Program supported by the California Department of Public Health, reports that for women in their program who achieved a prepregnancy A1c of less than 7 percent, the rate of anomalies was only 1.4 percent. Of women who enrolled in the program after their first trimester, however, 11 percent had babies with abnormalities.

The risk of congenital abnormalities among the babies of diabetic women is locked into a close correlation with blood sugar control at the time of conception. An A1c less than 7 percent carries no increased risk of abnormalities. With an A1c between 7.2 and 8.1 percent, the risk of abnormalities jumps to 14 percent. For A1c's between 8.2 and 11.1 percent, the risk is an appalling 23 percent, and for greater than 11.2 percent, the risk rises to greater than 25 percent. That's more than a one in four chance of a tragedy that could have been avoided.

Cheryl Alkon, author of *Balancing Pregnancy with Pre-existing Diabetes* says:

> *I moved back to Massachusetts to live with my boyfriend, and picked a new endocrinologist to follow me for regular diabetes care. The endocrinologist I picked was seeing new patients, but spent most of her time seeing pregnancy patients (she is the head of the pregnancy and diabetes program at the medical center near me). So, while I saw her as a nonpregnant patient at first, I knew I would work with her when I began thinking about pregnancy. After I got married, I met with her as a patient who was trying to conceive. It took me a good year to get pregnant, and I saw her every 6 weeks in the pregnancy clinic with the mindset of keeping my A1c under 7 that whole time.*

Brandy Barnes, RN, CDE, the founder of DiabetesSisters, spent days, months and even years planning for a *high-risk* pregnancy:

> *I read books, got my A1c to a respectable level of 6.0, reduced my caffeine consumption, and interviewed high-risk obstetricians, virtually everything I could think of . . . Nonetheless, it was about three months into my pregnancy when I realized the critical component I had overlooked. I searched high and low for a woman with diabetes who had experienced pregnancy and could answer my questions . . . or just tell me what I was going through was normal, and came up empty handed.*
>
> *Experiencing pregnancy for the first time as a young woman is scary enough, but having diabetes adds another level of unknown variables to the picture. When insulin requirements are increasing daily (reaching double or triple your prepregnancy amount), you really want someone who has experienced it to tell you, "I've been there and done that and know how scary it is."*
>
> *Having support from a woman with diabetes would have allowed me to relax and enjoy my pregnancy so much more. I would have been able to focus on the really important things rather than spending time worrying about unnecessary fears.*

Brandy's realization was the impetus behind the creation of Diabetes Sisters (www.diabetessisters.org), an international nonprofit organization dedicated to the needs of women with diabetes.

Not everything in life can be planned however.

Stella Biggs went off the pill right before she headed on a vacation to Europe with her husband:

> *We figured this might be our only chance to go to Europe for a while if we did start a family soon. I had talked to my endocrinologist and was prepared with my A1c being in range (in the 6.0 to 6.5 range) and then went off the pill. Of course, Europe was so romantic that we came home with our "European souvenir" and it only took about 2 months of being off the pill. Thank goodness, I never tried that before! I did not know I was pregnant until the end of my first trimester, and I had been drinking wine in Europe, going on roller coasters, etc., while I was pregnant. As soon as I had figured out there was something wrong, I was pleasantly surprised that it did not take long, but regretful for the wine, etcetera. Obviously, I changed my habits right away.*

In *The Diabetic Woman, All Your Questions Answered*, Dr. Lois Jovanovic says, "It's so much easier to plan to have a baby by first getting your blood sugars as close to normal as possible, rather than having to play catch-up by manipulating insulin, diet, and exercise to quickly normalize blood sugars so your baby does not experience high blood sugars." She recommends that women who are planning on becoming pregnant should "pretend they are pregnant." She also said that it's important to interview your physicians, "Find an OB who has seen at least 5 type 1 diabetic women in the last year. You want a physician who really knows," and that women may have to travel to find high-risk doctors to meet their needs.

■ Work to get an A1c of 7.0 or lower when you begin planning for pregnancy.
■ Meet with your diabetes and pregnancy team. This can include an endocrinologist, nutritionist, educator, and ob-gyn.
■ Start taking folic acid.
■ Tests: Rubella, complications, and so forth.

EDUCATION

Preparing for a diabetic pregnancy is like preparing for a marathon. When Laura Bennett, a type 1 diabetic, mother of three and a pregnancy blogger for Diabetes Sisters, began training for her first marathon, she read everything she could to educate herself about distance running. Laura also found running partners for support and practiced running a little further each week until the race day. When Laura decided to become pregnant, she said, "If I can complete a marathon, I can get through this pregnancy." She was in great physical shape, and her blood sugars were in good control because of her running, however, "Finding information on type 1 diabetes and pregnancy was difficult. Almost everything I came across was about gestational diabetes or type 2 [diabetes]. Sometimes, the information I did find was so discouraging and frightening that I thought, maybe, I shouldn't risk it and just adopt. Luckily, my endocrinologist was very supportive and I found the most amazing OB."

NUTRITION

When healthy eating becomes a habit in the planning stage, it will be easier to maintain during pregnancy. Dr. Liz Stephens recommends that you have a nutritionist and/or diabetes educator to work with who "can help with nutritional suggestions and get away from the standard pregnancy meal-snack-meal-snack that is so tricky with type 1 diabetes—thinking outside the box is [the] key!" Lyndsay Riffe, RD, CDE, LDN (who is also a type 1 diabetic), says, "Women who desire to become pregnant and are overweight can benefit from weight loss prior to conceiving." Any changes to diet should be approved by a doctor. Lyndsay recommends:

1. Focusing on high fiber foods (whole grains, fruits, vegetables, and beans), packing lunches and snacks from home to take to work, and avoid carbohydrate overloading. Balance and consistency are tools to get your sugar under control.
2. Keep your personal glycemic index, if you know eating grapes makes your blood sugar spike, avoid grapes. Diabetes is not a one-size-fits-all lifestyle.

3. Meet with a registered dietician (RD) or RD with certified diabetes educator (CDE). See http://www.eatright.org or www.diabeteseducators .org to find a local dietician and help separating fact from fiction.

EXERCISE

Exercise needs and abilities change during pregnancy, but getting 30 minutes of exercise at least five times a week is more important now than ever. Laura Bennett decreased the intensity of her runs before she became pregnant, but maintained a consistent, low-impact, exercise routine to keep her blood sugars balanced. As always, it's important to talk to your doctor about exercise when you are planning a pregnancy.

As a mother of three, Laura Bennett says that exercise is important to her life and diabetes management, but was even more imperative when she was pregnant:

> *Getting ready to have a baby when you have type 1 diabetes is hard work, but I found that exercise was so helpful. A few months before I decided to try to get pregnant with my first baby, I trained for and completed a marathon. (A little extreme, I know, but I enjoyed running and thought that completing such a difficult task would help prepare me both physically and mentally for a pregnancy, and it did!) Obviously, not everyone needs to run a marathon or anything close to that before becoming pregnant, but I do think having exercise as a regular part of your routine before becoming pregnant is so important.*
>
> *Keeping "perfect" blood sugars while pregnant is difficult, if not impossible sometimes! But here is where exercise was so useful. It helps your body use insulin more effectively; it can help with those postmeal peaks, give you more energy, and bring down a high blood sugar more quickly than insulin alone. There is nothing like the panic of seeing a blood sugar reading that is over 200 [mg/dl] when you are pregnant. My mind would immediately remember all those horror stories I had heard, and I*

couldn't help but imagine the damage my high blood sugar was doing to my poor innocent baby trying to grow inside my sugary body. (Ah, the guilt of pregnancy and diabetes!) That feeling of powerlessness was overwhelming as I would wait for a blood sugar to come down. In order to more quickly lower a blood sugar, I would often do some kind of exercise: walking, jumping jacks (before my belly had grown too much), weights, etcetera . . . anything to get my heart rate up so my blood sugar would come down.

I tried to do some form of exercise at least four times a week. In the beginning of my first pregnancy, I ran through the first and into the second trimester. I didn't run for as hard or as long as I did before I was pregnant, but I did continue running until my growing belly made it uncomfortable. After that, I walked. I was able to walk through all three of my pregnancies up until I delivered. I am convinced that I was able to recover from each delivery quickly because of the exercise I had done while pregnant.

After my daughter was born, I continued to walk and would push her in the stroller. I walked during my second and third pregnancies, mostly because I wasn't a fan of running and pushing a jogger. I am now pushing all three of my kiddos around, and dragging our dog on walks too. It is quite the ordeal, and we load up on plenty of snacks for the kids and me, because one thing I didn't ever want was to have a low while exercising. It's too scary to be in the middle of a run or walk and realize I'm low, so I always check before I leave the house and always carry some glucose tabs, a juice box, or a granola bar, just in case.

GESTATIONAL DIABETES MELLITUS

Gestational diabetes mellitus (GDM) affects about 4 percent of all pregnant women—about 135,000 cases of gestational diabetes in the United States each year.

At Risk

- Women with a parent, brother, or sister with diabetes
- African American, American Indian, Asian American, Hispanic/Latino, or Pacific Island women
- Women who are 25 years old or older
- Women who are overweight
- Women who have had gestational diabetes before or have given birth to at least one baby weighing more than 9 pounds
- Women who have been told that they have "prediabetes," a condition in which blood glucose levels are higher than normal but not yet high enough for a diagnosis of diabetes. Other names for it are "impaired glucose tolerance" and "impaired fasting glucose."
- Women who have checked any of these risk factors, ask your health care team about testing for gestational diabetes

High Risk
You are at high risk if you are overweight, have had gestational diabetes before, have a strong family history of diabetes, or have glucose in your urine. If you are at high risk, your blood glucose level may be checked at your first prenatal visit. If your test results are normal, you will be checked again sometime between weeks 24 and 28 of your pregnancy.

Average Risk
You are at average risk if you have one or more of the risk factors mentioned previously. If you have an average risk for gestational diabetes, you will be tested sometime between weeks 24 and 28 of pregnancy.

Low Risk
You are at low risk if you do not have any of the risk factors mentioned previously. If you are at low risk, your doctor may decide that you do not need to be checked.

According to the CDC, women with GDM have a 25–45 percent higher risk for recurrence in the next pregnancy and a future risk of nongestational diabetes (primarily, type 2 diabetes) ranging from 17–63 percent during the 5–16 years following the index pregnancy.

Effects of Gestational Diabetes on the Baby

Untreated or uncontrolled gestational diabetes can mean problems for your baby, such as:

■ Being born very large and with extra fat; this can make delivery difficult and more dangerous for your baby
■ Low blood glucose right after birth
■ Breathing problems

If you have gestational diabetes, your health care team may recommend some extra tests to check on your baby, such as:

■ An ultrasound exam to see how your baby is growing
■ *Kick counts* to check your baby's activity (the time between the baby's movements) or special *stress* tests

Working closely with your health care team will help you give birth to a healthy baby. Both you and your baby are at an increased risk for type 2 diabetes for the rest of your lives.

Effects of Gestational Diabetes on the Mother

Often, women with gestational diabetes have no symptoms. However, gestational diabetes may:

■ Increase your risk of high blood pressure during pregnancy
■ Increase your risk of a large baby and the need for cesarean section at delivery

The good news is that your gestational diabetes will probably go away after your baby is born. However, you will be more likely to get type 2 diabetes later in your life. (See the information on how to lower your chances of getting type 2 diabetes.) You may also get gestational diabetes if you get pregnant again.

Some women wonder whether breastfeeding is okay after they have had gestational diabetes. Breastfeeding is recommended for most babies, including those whose mothers had gestational diabetes.

Treatment for Gestational Diabetes

- A healthy, low-carb meal plan
- Physical activity
- Insulin (if needed)

Blood glucose targets for most women with gestational diabetes:

- Fasting: ,95 mg/dl
- 1 hour after meal: <140 mg/dl
- 2 hours after meal: <120 mg/dl

Women will probably have a blood glucose test 6–12 weeks after their baby is born to see whether they still have diabetes though most women will not. They are, however, at risk for having gestational diabetes during future pregnancies or getting type 2 diabetes later.

Rebecca Walter Bryant was diagnosed with gestational diabetes during her third pregnancy. She says:

I was just about to be 35 when we were attempting to have our third child. I had no fears about this as I have had no real health issues with any other pregnancy. We were very excited to try to have a daughter. So, we started planning our third pregnancy a little over a year after the birth of our second son. We wanted these two to be close in age, and within 8 more months, I was pregnant. I was tested for blood sugar irregularities at my 28th week appointment, as was typical for expectant mothers over the age of 35. I failed the test. I was sent for further, more detailed testing, that did come back positive for gestational diabetes. After drinking 75 grams of glucose, my blood glucose (BG) came back over 280 mg/dl.

From there, I had to take a crash course in diabetes from how to manage my care to checking my blood sugars daily. I had to learn the complications that could arise if I did not adhere to a strict diet, take prescribed medication, and follow weight-gain requirements. For the first time, someone else's life was totally dependent on me.

My ob-gyn was trained as a high-risk physician and he became my primary care physician handling my diabetes care during the pregnancy. Since I had gestational diabetes, everyone assumed that the diabetes would go away once I had delivered my daughter. I was sent to diabetic nutrition class at my local hospital and was taught how to count carbs and learn correct portion control. I was also sent to a diabetes educator who showed me how to use a blood glucose meter, test strips, and put me at ease when it came to learning to check my BG. I really was starting from scratch. I knew nothing about diabetes.

Since I was considered high risk *due to my advanced maternal age and diabetes, I was monitored more often than in my prior pregnancies. I studied diabetes like a college student and wanted to care for my unborn child as well as possible. I took the issue very seriously, as the complications of not doing so were made very clear to me. For example, in my previous pregnancies, I ate whatever I wanted. Once I learned how to eat properly, as advised by a nutritionist, I can say that I really did follow most of their directions. I can recall eating a snack: 1 carb, 1 protein, 1 fat. I believe, in hindsight, that I was good about 90 percent of the time. I think I was rewarded with a healthier weight gain and fewer complications.*

I managed stress during pregnancy by continuing to exercise and by educating myself. I recall getting every book I could find on gestational diabetes and trying to learn all I could about taking care of myself. I think being an informed patient made a huge difference in my stress, because I could make decisions that would positively affect the outcome of my pregnancy. I also made sure to get a lot of rest and even took naps at work when I had a break and my body needed a rest. I also started journaling at that time, a habit, which I still have today. Writing things down has been great therapy for me, and keeping a food and BG journal has been instrumental in keeping me on track.

I will admit that I didn't know how much work diabetes would be. I had to learn to take the best possible care of myself for the remainder of the pregnancy, and that at the end, I would be rewarded with a healthy baby and get my life and health back in the end. (This of course, did not happen.)

My daughter was gaining a lot of weight toward the end of the pregnancy and my ob-gyn was concerned of me delivering a 10-pound child. I was induced at 39 weeks. I had what I call a "MASH Unit" of at least 10 people surrounding me in the delivery room, and no one, except my husband was allowed in the room. These people consisted of two teams, one for me, and one for my daughter. It was like nothing I had ever seen before. Once she was delivered, I got to see her but not hold her. She was 9 pounds 9 ounces, and they had to rush her to [neonatal intensive care unit] NICU to put her on a little insulin pump as soon as she was born. I didn't even get to hold her. That made the situation scarier than it really turned out to be.

She turned out to be fine after 2 days, and we were able to go home on the third day. She has had no signs of blood sugar problems since her birth 5 years ago.

One thing that I would like people to take away from my story is that I kept being told over and over again, "the diabetes will go away after your child is delivered." I kept wondering, how does this happen? I was told that the sugar issues are carried with the placenta and once the [baby] was delivered the issues would go away.

I think all gestational diabetic patients are told that the rate of acquiring type 2 diabetes in the future is increased by something like 20 percent depending on the patient. If they eat unhealthy food and gain a lot of weight, then the diabetes is likely to come back. I always had this in my mind. I knew I was going to have to be on watch for symptoms in the future and be proactive with my health.

After my last pregnancy, I never felt the same again. I continued to check my fasting blood sugars, postpregnancy, in the mornings or after exercise when I felt weird. I had to find a general physician who said, "Yes, it does look like you have diabetes," but he could not tell me how to properly treat myself or what kind of diabetes I had. It took me a year of feeling weird and questioning my health in order to get to an endocrinologist who diagnosed me as LADA, latent autoimmune diabetes in adults. She took very good care of me, especially since I was not the typical patient she came by in her practice. She cared that I was a young mother with two babies at home to care for. She taught me a lot, and I owe her a debt of gratitude to this day for providing me with answers to all of my questions.

I am now essentially a type 1 diabetic, and I have been insulin dependent for over 3 years now. I chose to have my tubes tied and then had a hysterectomy for other issues several years ago. I had planned no more children after going through the issues of my 3rd pregnancy. I am doing fine today and know that I have to take my diabetes care seriously and start fresh with it every day. If I want to live a long, healthy life for these children that I brought in to this world, then I have to be mindful of my treatment and my on-going care.

FIRST TRIMESTER

The first trimester can be almost a honeymoon stage of diabetes. Many women will have decreased insulin needs and frequent low blood sugar levels.

Many women find it extremely challenging to maintain optimal blood glucose levels in this early stage of pregnancy as their bodies are undergoing so many hormonal and physical changes. Women with type 2 diabetes are advised to discuss their medication with their diabetes team. Some women with type 2 will need to switch from diabetes tablets to insulin injections during pregnancy. Insulin needs for women with type 1 diabetes often decrease in the early stages of pregnancy—between

6 weeks' and 16 weeks' gestation. This is dangerous because it can cause severe low blood sugars to occur, sometimes without warning. Preventing a hypo is better than treating one.

TIPS

1. Check if you have a GlucaGen prescription and current supply, and make sure that your partner knows how to use it!
2. Carry glucose tabs or sweets in your handbag, glove box, and sports bag at all times.
3. Make a plan with your team to coordinate the times and number of blood glucose tests you do each day or week.

Kristin Makszin says that one of her biggest challenges has been comparing herself to other pregnant women. She says:

> *The emotional burden of blood sugar maintenance is my biggest challenge. My blood sugars have been awesome— but I still find myself almost constantly worried about what they are.*
>
> *I also find it very difficult and counterproductive to compare my pregnancy with the experience of nondiabetic women. Many women talk about the joys and challenges of pregnancy. For me, they are just a reminder of how different pregnancy is with preexisting diabetes. I have found that I need the diabetes online community now, more than ever, to connect with women who had pregnancies like mine.*
>
> *When women tell me about funny cravings they had, I think that I don't have the luxury to crave things that don't fit into my diet. So I don't. But I prefer to avoid reminders of how my pregnancy is different.*

SECOND TRIMESTER

Late in the second trimester, a woman's insulin requirements will begin to increase. This is caused by the release of hormones from the placenta. These hormones decrease the effectiveness of insulin. Make sure that you tell your doctor or nurse when blood sugars are above normal (95 mg/dl fasting or 120 mg/dl 2 hours after meals) for 3 days in a row, or if they are often less than 60 mg/dl. Around 20 weeks' gestation, most women will begin to need more insulin. Continued blood sugar monitoring and insulin adjustments are necessary to prevent high blood sugars. An average weight gain of about 9 pounds is expected in this trimester.[3]

Cheryl Alkon has diabetic retinopathy and says, "I had laser treatment three times during my first pregnancy and twice during my second. This was to prevent my retinopathy from advancing during pregnancy, rather than a response to eye problems themselves. (My vision is clear and [has] never changed during the pregnancy)."

According to CDC, "In the reproductive years, diabetic nephropathy may be diagnosed somewhat earlier in women than men because as many as 25 percent of all cases of diabetic nephropathy among women can be diagnosed during pregnancy. In early pregnancy, women with preexisting diabetic nephropathy may have a marked increase in protein excretion because of the rise in glomerular filtration rate that normally occurs in pregnancy. This phenomenon may increase the likelihood of earlier detection of diabetic nephropathy."

THIRD TRIMESTER

All the vital organs are fully formed in the third trimester. The baby's bones, especially in the head, are soft and flexible. Your baby will now begin to gain more weight and grow rapidly. At the end of the seventh month, your baby will weigh 2 ½-3 pounds and will be 14-17 inches long. By the time your baby is ready to be delivered, he or she should weigh about 7 ¼-7 ½ pounds and should be close to 20 inches long.

Because of the release of hormones and other substances from the placenta, those who are taking insulin may require two to three times their pre-pregnancy dosage. During the last 2 months of pregnancy, your doctor will evaluate the growth and development of your baby and talk with you about the best method of delivery. The frequency of doctor visits will increase to once a week. Continue to bring a log book to each doctor or clinic visit. Because of the great strides in diabetes care for pregnant women, many mothers are now able to carry their babies full term and deliver vaginally. If your baby is too large to be delivered safely vaginally, a cesarean section will be a necessary method of delivery.[4]

In my third trimester, as my baby and its pancreas grew, I became increasingly insulin resistant. I had to give myself larger doses of insulin to cover the foods I was eating and had to find food that wouldn't raise my blood sugar. I was tired of eggs for breakfast! I remember going to the doctor every 2 weeks, so frequently that I knew all the parking attendants and the names of the women behind the check in desk. I had to keep detailed records of my blood sugars and exercise for my doctor's review. I had to test my blood sugars at least ten times a day, and the tips of my fingers were hardened like the calluses that form on the bottom of your feet in the summer.

The third trimester is the hard part. I'd been there twice before, so I remembered the work, the large doses of insulin, and the constant testing; and I knew it would all be over soon. I knew that all the hard work would provide our baby with a healthy environment to grow and become strong, but still, there are moments when I wanted to scream in frustration, moments when I wanted to curl up in my bed and sleep for weeks, wake up in a new body, moments like this when I wanted to feel sorry for myself and then, it was finally over.

FOURTH TRIMESTER

Birth

Dr. Jovanovic says that women with diabetes can have a natural and normal delivery through excellent blood sugar management.

I had hoped for natural births with my own children, but after a difficult labor, I had to have an emergency cesarean section with our first born and two more cesareans followed. I'd always imagined my experience would be like my mom's and that I would have stories to share with my boys just like the story that she told me every year on my birthday.

On the evening of January 19, 1971, my mom and dad were in a grocery store in suburban Boston. It was a frigidly cold night, and mom remembers walking through the aisles when suddenly, a rush of liquid spilled between her legs. She says that as she searched for my dad, her shoes squeaked with water. (This part of the story always reminds me of a camping trip in fourth grade when we hiked up a river in our sneakers. I liked the way the water squished out of my shoes each time I put a foot down and the sound that my foot made when I pulled it up again to take another step.) Mom and Dad hurried home and began counting contractions.

When it was time to go to the hospital, my dad went outside to start the car, an MG, a gift to my mother from her father—a car that was entirely impractical in the middle of a New England winter. By the time that dad brought mom outside, the car was dead. It was the middle of the night, and they had to call a friend who drove recklessly along the icy streets to the Newton-Wellesley Hospital. When she was safe inside, mom practiced her Lamaze breathing. My parents were young hippies. Dad was the first husband allowed in the delivery room of the hospital. Mom refused any pain medication, and then 5 hours later, I was born, a perfect 10 on the APGAR scale.

My mother has told me the story of my birth ever since I was a young girl. Even though I am nearing 40 years old, I look forward every year to hearing my birth story. The details of that cold night, the dead car, my mother's refusal of pain medication, and my father's inclusion in the delivery room were all dramatic and romantic. Each year, I am always surprised to discover something that I didn't know before.

My children's birth stories are different. I didn't experience the surprise of my water breaking naturally or the surge of nervous excitement that follows. I didn't count contractions. With our first son, my water was formally broken in the hospital and my labor was induced with Pitocin. After hours of pushing, vacuuming, and forceps, I was rushed into the surgery room and our baby was finally delivered through cesarean section.

I want to continue the birth story tradition that my mother began, but as I cuddle with Will or Miles on the eve of their birthdays, I find myself at a loss for words. Lying next to them in bed, I see myself in the passenger seat of our car as Dale and I drive to the hospital. I see us checking into labor and delivery, my arm getting poked with IVs, and the constant presence of nurses checking my blood sugars. I see myself being numbed with a spinal block. I see a curtain being drawn over my face so I won't be able to see my internal organs, but I can't tell this story to my children. I don't like the words available to me like *cesarean* and *high risk*, and I struggle with "you were born" or "you were delivered" or "you were cut from my body." I find myself hurrying through the memories and wondering if my sons are bored by their cold and clinical-sounding birth stories.

When Reid was born, I thought it would be different, I considered myself experienced at the whole diabetic birthing thing. But I realize now, almost 2 years later, that each birth is different, and they were all perfect in some ways and frustrating in others. After Reid was born, on the third day in the hospital, a young nurse took my newborn son away from me. She said, "You shouldn't be holding the baby when your blood sugar is so low."

Reid and I were alone in the room when the nurse came. I'd pressed the call button because my blood sugar was dropping, and I didn't have any juice. Dale was at home with the boys; they were not coming to visit for another hour, and I could feel myself going down. When I tested my blood sugar, the meter read 37 mg/dl. My hands were shaking, and it felt like I was slipping. I needed help and was irritated because if I'd been at home, I could have gone to the fridge for juice. But I wasn't home, I was alone with my newborn son in the hospital. My blood sugar was precariously low, and I was being asked to let go of my baby, to hand him over to someone else who could keep him safe, because he wasn't safe with me.

I felt small and helpless. I felt guilty too, guilty for getting low, guilty for having this high risk body, and guilty for handing over my son to someone more capable. But I know better than to beat myself up over this disease. So I will continue the family tradition of telling birth stories to my sons because I love hearing my own. I will tell them the truth about the hard work, the risks, and the mistakes that are a part of being a woman with a chronic illness; I am the mother now, and this is my story.

BREASTFEEDING

I am proud of the fact that I have breastfed all three of my children for longer than a year, but I also know that breastfeeding is not for everyone, whether you are a woman with diabetes or not. Breastfeeding got easier each time, and I am now in the process of weaning our son Reid who is 18 months old, because we are both ready. Nursing is another one of those areas where myths and a general lack of information exacerbate fear or worry and some mothers may not even try as a result.

The CDC report states:

> *Women with type 1 diabetes choose to breast-feed at the same rate as mothers from the general hospital population; however, mothers with type 1 diabetes are more likely to add formula supplements within several weeks of delivery. In addition, the onset of copious milk production is delayed among women with type 1 diabetes. The extent*

of the delay in lactogenesis correlates directly with adequacy of maternal glycemic control. Once lactation is established, the breast milk of women with type 1 diabetes does not differ in lactose, protein, lipid, or calcium content, but it may contain higher levels of glucose and sodium and lower concentrations of long-chain polyunsaturated fatty acids. Data on any effects of these qualitative differences in breast milk are not presently available.

Cheryl Alkon struggled to breastfeed her first son:

This time (my daughter is 8 weeks), I am happy to say that I am nursing her, though she has been a slow weight gainer and while she's a great nurser, I have had to pump breast milk regularly as well as supplement with formula (though less than I had to for my son) for her to stay on the weight gain curve.

For my son, nursing was a frustrating endeavor in that I would nurse him for what seemed like hours, and he'd always be hungry and screaming afterwards. Then I'd pump milk and feed it to him, and then feed him formula. This [is] despite [of] meeting with two lactation consultants, taking all kinds of milk-producing herbs and meds, and educating myself on every aspect of breastfeeding and low milk supply. Finally, I just dropped the nursing after about a month and pumped [milk] for 8.5 months and fed him formula the rest of the time. I really wanted to give him as much breast milk as possible for the health benefits and really researched what kind of formula would be best for him. I went with a hydrolyzed formula, which has broken-down cow's protein in it; researchers in the [Trial to Reduce Insulin-dependent diabetes mellitus in the Genetically at Risk] TRIGR study are finding that this is less likely to trigger a type 1 diabetes diagnosis than intact cow's milk formula has. I have since talked to the researcher doing this work for my book (long after my son was off formula entirely) who confirmed my theory; this made me calmer about having to feed my kids formula since I couldn't produce enough to exclusively feed them [with] breast milk alone.

STATISTICS

■ A 2006 study of more than 15,000 children, published in Diabetes Care, showed that breastfeeding does a better job of preventing obesity in children of diabetic mothers.
■ Breastfeeding may reduce the risks of developing diabetes.

Breastfeeding Postdelivery

■ Your baby will be tested for low blood glucose within the first 24 hours after birth, and it needs to be above 2.5 mmol/L. The baby may have produced extra insulin to compensate for excess glucose, from his or her mother, passing across the placenta during the pregnancy. The baby's pancreas usually needs 24-48 hours to adapt and return to normal insulin production.
■ Breastfeeding within 30-60 minutes of birth can reduce the risk of your baby experiencing low blood glucose levels. Consistent nursing on the first day will also assist your baby to maintain blood glucose levels above 2.5 mmol/L. Blood glucose that are below these levels for an extended period may affect a baby's brain development.

TIPS IN BREASTFEEDING

■ Breastfeeding takes a lot of energy. Be ready to convert your insulin doses back to the amount you were on before the pregnancy, and make sure you understand the potential blood glucose changes.
■ Set up a comfortable area where you will sit to feed your baby, with snacks on hand in case you feel low.
■ Test your blood glucose before and after a nursing session to see how your levels drop.
■ Dr. Jovanovic strongly advises sitting in a rocking chair (or with a pillow on the floor in the nursery) to nurse during the night.

She says that low blood sugars are too much of a risk to nurse with your baby in bed next to you.

■ Eat healthy and frequent snacks, breastfeeding uses extra calories that need to be replaced.

Benefits to Moms
■ Helps new moms take extra weight off
■ Endorphins are released
■ For women who had gestational diabetes, breastfeeding can decrease the risks of developing type 2 diabetes later in life

If you don't have your baby with you, ask your midwife about expressing within the first 4 hours of your baby's birth. Your breasts make milk on a supply and demand basis. If you express milk from your breasts, they will keep producing milk for your baby.

If you plan not to breastfeed for long, just 6–8 weeks of breastfeeding gives many benefits to your baby, including immunity from certain types of infections.

The initiation of breast milk or "milk coming in" (usually on day 3) may be delayed for 24–48 hours in some women with type 1 diabetes. Because your blood glucose levels may fall rapidly during and following breastfeeding, just like any other physical activity, you may need to:

■ Snack prior to or while breastfeeding such as fruits, crackers, or sandwiches.
■ Treat yourself immediately should a "hypo" occur.
■ Stay hydrated.
■ Develop a routine for feeding your baby, so you are able to have your meals on time and reduce your risk of hypos.
■ Rub expressed milk into your nipples after each feed to help prevent nipple soreness and heal cracked nipples.
■ Test your blood glucose after a feed, especially during the night, to avoid nocturnal hypos.
■ If you are having trouble with breastfeeding or your baby is losing weight, is continuously unsettled, or has few soaked diapers, phone your hospital's lactation midwife for advice anytime, even though your baby is already born.

- Talk to your team about setting new blood glucose goals and insulin adjustments during breastfeeding.
- Talk to your midwife about successful breastfeeding strategies. Ask about storing breast milk to complement feeds if necessary.

POSTPARTUM DEPRESSION

A study conducted by researchers at the Harvard Medical School have shown that "Pregnant women and new mothers with diabetes had nearly double the risk of developing postpartum depression as women without diabetes, a new study reports, revealing a potential risk factor for a serious psychological disorder that affects more than one in 10 new mothers."

Researchers said that the stress of managing a chronic illness might contribute to the risk of depression.

Opting for Adoption

Choosing pregnancy is not for every woman. Rachel Garlinghouse and her husband chose not to have children biologically:

> *It was a year after my diagnosis that we decided we were ready to start a family, but I knew that my body wasn't ready for a pregnancy. I was still adjusting to life with diabetes. We talked, prayed, and researched, and decided to adopt. In November of 2008, we adopted a baby girl, Ella. Then in November of 2010, we adopted again, another baby girl, whom we named Emery. Adoption isn't the same as having biological children, but it can be equally as wonderful. Without diabetes, we probably wouldn't have adopted, so as crazy as it sounds, diabetes was a blessing. I cannot imagine my life without my daughters. I'm often asked, "So you don't want your own kids?" My daughters are my own. I don't wake up every morning and think about the fact that they were adopted. We get up in the morning and go about our day like any other family. Yes, adoption has its own unique challenges and opportunities, but at the end of the day, my girls are mine, and I am theirs.*

I had many fears about pregnancy because I did my research; I knew there were numerous potential complications. I honestly feel that not many people I talked to (diabetic or not) understood the seriousness and dangers of pregnancy while managing type 1 diabetes. Granted, I was only 1 year into my diagnosis when we were ready to start a family. I knew my diabetes wasn't predictable enough at that point to have a biological child, so we chose adoption. Rather than let diabetes decide for us when we could start a family, we decided to take charge and adopt.

My doctor told me, at the point in which my A1c came down to a healthy number, to go ahead and get pregnant. He recommended that I do so [while] young (before age 30) to have the healthiest pregnancy possible. I'm glad I didn't decide to have biological children at that point, because soon after my honeymoon period (meaning with my diabetes) ended my sugar skyrocketed. I struggled for a year to get them back under control. Think what those highs and lows could have done to my baby and/or me!

Some agencies only allow infertile couples to adopt, and we didn't have an infertility diagnosis. So we were somewhat limited in which agency we could use. The first agency we used required a letter from my endocrinologist. All adoptive couples are required to have a physical for the adoption to demonstrate that they are physically healthy enough to care for a child.

When we finalized Ella's adoption, Ella's guardian ad litem did ask me some questions about my diabetes in court. I had nothing to hide. I work really hard to be healthy.

I was afraid that no birth couple or birth mom would want us to adopt her child because we didn't have the traditional adoption story—infertility. But obviously, that wasn't an issue.

Pregnancy isn't for everyone; adoption isn't for everyone. Do a lot of research and don't be afraid to be confident in your educated decision. A lot of people questioned why we didn't want "our own" children. I took that as an opportunity to explain that diabetes impacts each patient differently, and for me, a pregnancy wasn't healthy or safe. I was also able to educate others on adoption. My daughters are "my own" children. Adoption was our number one choice (not "second best"), and we have been blessed with two beautiful daughters. We did consider surrogacy; however, there are many medical risks associated with harvesting a woman's eggs and additionally, I had many ethical concerns with the entire process. Surrogacy is legally, medically, emotionally, and ethically complicated. In the end, we knew in our hearts that having children who shared our genes wasn't important to us. What mattered is that we became parents.

AUTHENTIC ADVICE

■ Rachel Garlinghouse says:
A biological child just wasn't the right choice for us at the point in which we were ready to grow our family. (In fact, I really admire the women who face a pregnancy with diabetes; I can imagine it's a full time job to manage blood sugars even more strictly than ever before). I am all about self-education and making educated, confident decisions. Each woman with diabetes is in a unique place in her life, and we shouldn't judge one another for the decisions we make regarding how to build our families or manage our disease.

■ Cara Bauer says:
A diabetic pregnancy is hard work. It requires you to be diligent about blood sugar control, constantly testing and staying on top of your blood sugars. You're in need of more doc[tor] visits and tests. But our diet is probably a big help, we're more likely to eat healthier foods because of the diabetes. But it can be done. If you're up for the work, the payoff at the end with a healthy baby is so worth it. I would not change a thing about

my pregnancies, deliveries, and children. They were worth every moment I drove myself nuts during pregnancy.

- Stella Biggs says:

  There are so many blogs from [people with] type 1 [diabetes] who went through pregnancy, and there are even books to read. Make sure you check out those sites before you get pregnant. I would definitely not think that Steel Magnolias is going to happen to you! There are so many [people with] type 1 [diabetes] that have had healthy and beautiful pregnancies and children. It does take work, but the reward is worth it!

Becoming a mother was a turning point for me. My body was transformed from something broken, something in need of constant medical attention to a giver of life. I have never felt more beautiful or strong than when I was pregnant (parts of the pregnancy anyway). A decade of my life was spent pregnant or nursing and caring for babies. When I look back on my 30s, I can see that I emerged as a changed woman, a woman with confidence who has a better appreciation of the strength within.

10   Motherhood

Becoming a mother was a motivation to take care of my diabetes. For the first time in my life, I wanted to take care of myself so I could be a strong and healthy mom for my children. I remember a time when our first son, Will, was still a baby, and I was at home alone with him. I was a new mother, new to staying at home and being isolated from the rest of the world, but I loved it. I was also somewhat new to nursing and was still trying to figure out how to manage blood sugars. Every morning, I took Will out in the jogger for my daily run. I pushed him through the neighborhood for 30 minutes, which helped me maintain my sanity and, after frequent sleepless nights, helped to wake me up a little.

One warm spring morning, we returned home from our run, and I lingered outside with Will and stretched. He was just learning to walk and I let him toddle up and back on the sidewalk in front of our house. He was having a great time and didn't want to come in, but I could feel my blood sugar begin to drop. For some reason, it dropped quickly that day, and I remember looking at the house and thinking that I needed to get back there. I needed to get to the kitchen, but I had to stay with Will and the kitchen seemed so far away. Something inside of me knew that I shouldn't pick him up but my mind was slowing down and I didn't know what to do. My legs started to shake and my vision flashed, but somehow, I picked my child up and stumbled the 100 yards to our house, up the stairs, and into the kitchen where I put him down on the floor crying. I then managed to open the fridge and pour orange juice down my throat. I felt like a horrible person, a failure as a mother, and when I looked at this small boy, I was sure he was scared of me.

That happened 10 years ago and I'd like to say that I've never gotten low with my kids since but that would be a lie. Of course, I have and of course I will again. It doesn't happen often, less often in fact ever since

I became a mother, but it still happens. And now that my children are older (Will is 10, Miles is 7, and Reid is 2), they know what to do if I need help.

PLANNING A FAMILY

How many children make a family? I remember my ob-gyn telling me, "4 makes a family," after I gave birth to our second son Miles. When I became pregnant with Reid, almost 5 years later, it was a big surprise to us all. Are there different considerations for women with diabetes when it comes to family planning? I don't think so. I've had three successful pregnancies and three successful cesareans.

Michelle Sorensen has two daughters, aged 2 and 4 years, and is pregnant with twins—one boy and one girl. She says:

> *When I was diagnosed with diabetes at age 24, I remember an endocrinologist saying that it wouldn't be recommended that I have more than two pregnancies. However, after I had my second, my doctors would ask me whether I wanted a third, and said they didn't see any reason why I couldn't. My diabetes has been very well managed throughout my pregnancies, but of course it becomes harder to manage when life is busy. So my husband and I really debated the decision to have a third child, wanting to make sure that we could still prioritize my health and the overall health of our family.*

TALKING TO YOUR CHILDREN ABOUT DIABETES

Lisa Copen lives with rheumatoid arthritis and has written about parenting with chronic illness. She explains how to talk to your children about your diagnosis during the different developmental stages of childhood. "As a parent, if you become ill, your illness has a profound impact on the entire family system. In spite of your own increased stress, confusion, and anger, your children will look to you to maintain or return to normal family routines as soon as possible. If you, or your spouse, present an image of feeling overwhelmed or being consumed with the illness, your children will feel as if life is spiraling out of control.[1]

Infancy

The time of infancy is probably the easiest in terms of knowing how to respond. The primary developmental goal is to establish trust. The child is completely dependent on the mother (or primary caretakers) to have their basic physical and emotional needs met. With love and nurturing, the infant (and older baby) will thrive and grow.

Adults generally assume that a baby is too young or unaware to notice a change in a parent or family. However, infants and babies are extremely intuitive and can sense when a parent is upset or anxious. Any change in daily routine can throw a baby into a fretful state. When crisis occurs, you may see the following behaviors: increased crying and irritability, changes in appetite and sleep schedules, clinging behaviors, and regression. Separation anxiety, which occurs routinely, becomes exaggerated. Treat regressive behaviors casually and return to a normal routine as soon as possible.

If your toddler asks a question about your illness, answer openly and honestly. A rule of thumb is never offer more information than the child has requested. Concealing the illness or whispering about what is happening will not help. Children always suffer more from the tension of not knowing than from knowing the truth. Allowing the child to act out fears and frustration through play or art is also an excellent help.

Preschool

Preschool, ages 4–5 years, is the age of expansion. Preschoolers are ready to move out of the safety zone of the home and into a broader social arena. There is an increased reliance at this stage on *magical thinking*. To a preschooler, anything that happens, good or bad, is related to them and their behavior. If a parent becomes ill during this stage, the preschooler's view will be, "Mommy is sick because I told her she was mean."

In response to stress and change, preschoolers often present with extremes, either being all good or all bad. This is the child's attempt to maintain a sense of control and to feel less frightened. Regressive behaviors are likely to occur, especially with an increased reliance on a favorite security object (blanket, teddy bear, thumb-sucking).

To help preschoolers, it is essential to assure them that the illness is not their fault. Returning to a security object should be encouraged, rather than discouraged. Answer all questions honestly, including those about death. This is a good time to rely on books, which helps your child on working through complex and often frustrating feelings about illness.

School Age

The primary development goal of the *school-age stage* (6–10 years) is achievement.

The focus is school, outside activities, and developing strong peer relationships. Although the parents and the family are still central, the biggest concern is, "What will happen to me if you are ill?" This self-centeredness is normal. Although there is still some overlap with magical thinking, by the age of 8, children realize that illness may not be their fault. However, they are still not mature enough to remove themselves completely from the situation. The thinking now is: "If I'm good, mommy will feel better and things will be fine."

School-age children tend to show strong emotions in reaction to change. They may show anger at both parents: "Why did you let this happen?" They tend to have a lot of somatic complaints (headache, stomach pain, fatigue), especially when leaving for school. The child is often fearful to leave the ill parent; he or she often assumes a protective role. Earlier in this stage, children are fearful that if they leave, the parent may die. As such, preoccupation and fear of death may be common.

When attempting to help school-age children, it is important to recognize that angry outbursts are an attempt to grieve or release fearful feelings. The opposite reaction, denial, may also occur as the child hopes that the illness will just disappear. Children will have many more questions and concerns at this stage. However, only the simplest explanations need be given. Information that they don't understand will only frighten them and increase their anxiety. Questions about death must be answered directly. Evading questions leads to more fear.

Changes in school performance, either for better or worse, are common. It is essential to let the teachers know about the changes at home and to establish a feedback loop.

Adolescence

The final stage of development is *adolescence*. The primary goal is to develop a self-identity that is capable of independent action.

Adolescents work to achieve separation from parents and to become independent of the family system. This stage is a painful one for both parent and child, as both of them struggle in this journey toward separation.

Under normal circumstances, adolescents are known for their emotional volatility and moodiness. When a crisis occurs, you may see and hear even more expressions of anger, hurt, and confusion. The opposite extreme is also common—they may withdraw completely and not want to discuss your illness or their feelings about what's happening. There will be ambivalence about helping you. If you have an adolescent who is willing to do his or her part in helping the family, this will not extend outside the home. Fitting in and acceptance by peers will be much more important than appearing helpful to the family. It is normal for them to be embarrassed by the illness and not want to discuss it with friends or teachers.

This is an essential time for parents to fine tune their communication skills. It is imperative to listen to and understand the volatile outbursts of an adolescent. Accept these feelings without overreacting to their tone. Continue to set limits, rules, and boundaries, but keep the task of separation in mind. These outbursts are often fear-based.

At a time when they often feel out of control, teenagers cling to the hope that parents and family will remain structured and safe. Remember, even though he or she appears grown, your adolescent needs as much love and reassurance as your younger children. In discussions about your illness, be prepared to give much more detailed information, especially all the facts about the illness. A major concern or fear will be: "Will I get it too?"

Some adolescents (the withdrawing ones) may not want to hear about or discuss your illness. They may express anger or disappointment toward the ill parent. These behaviors serve to diffuse their own fears or feelings of inadequacy in controlling the changes that are occurring or may occur in the future. Honest and open discussion of your own feelings may help them to express their own feelings. One of the most difficult challenges for parents of the adolescent is to overcome the expectation that he or she will be mature enough to handle the situation and to provide support. In actuality, they are overburdened with their own concerns and too vulnerable to carry the additional adult concerns.

Cara Bauer says that her kids are well aware of her diabetes, and they understand to a point what needs to be done. She says, "They're sad I have diabetes, but they realize my routines with it keep me alive and healthy and here for them. They help me with snacks and such if I need it. A couple of times, my oldest daughter has needed to correct a kid who has made fun of diabetes, and I was very proud of her. I think my kids are more empathetic and patient because of it."

Cara says that her children have seen her get low and thinks that it is good for them to see that she's not perfect, and that sometimes, things happen that are out of our control. She says that the important part is learning to take responsibility.

Stella Biggs has two daughters, aged 7 and 5. She says that her daughters have seen the pump on her since the day they were born but didn't ask about it until they realized they didn't have one too. She says:

> *We didn't really talk about it until they started noticing the low blood sugars and could actually help me if I needed it. We told them, "mommy has a disease and that the pump helps her stay alive. She has to eat and check her blood sugar to keep her healthy." I'm not sure they really understand it yet, but eventually they will. Sometimes, they get mad at my diabetes, especially when we are heading to Disney and we have to wait until mommy's blood sugar goes up before we can go. They do get concerned, though, when "mommy gets silly." They know it is treatable and that I get better with juice, but I see the concern on their faces when I come back and they tell me they were scared. That just breaks my heart. I don't like to scare them, and I try my best not to scare them.*

Stella says that her girls have helped her before when her blood sugar drops. She says, "I don't think you are ever too young to learn to care for someone, not take care of them—but to really care."

BALANCING MOTHERHOOD AND DIABETES

As mothers with diabetes, sometimes, worrying about blood sugars or making sure what we eat, takes a back seat to the demands of our family. When the baby is crying, there's homework that needs to be done, there are laundries and chores, and it seems like there will never be enough time to do everything that needs to be done; then our blood sugar spikes, sometimes it feels like it's us against the world. There have been many days when I want to scream or cry in frustration, and diabetes is just one of the things that make my life harder. Those are the days that my grandmother's words ring in my head: "This too shall pass." I take a deep breath and hold on (or yell or figure out a way to go for a run or a walk), and it almost always gets better.

Rachel Garlinghouse has two young daughters, Ella and Emery and she says: "I know that if I do not put my health first, everyone in my family will suffer. Diabetes or not, how I treat myself is likely how my daughters will learn to treat themselves. I value exercise, healthy eating, sleep, and relaxation. I work very hard to make sure we aren't overscheduled as a family. At times, yes, it's difficult to say 'no' to others and 'yes' to self, but if you don't take care of yourself now, you will pay for it later."

Cara Bauer has three kids and says:

> *Aside from checking my blood sugar and having to deal with changing out my pump and such; for me, I don't think being a mom with diabetes is always much different from being a mom without it. I do need to realize my limitations in many things, I can't spontaneously go swimming with my kids, I need to do something with my pump. I need to keep on top of my blood sugars, but it only takes a few seconds. Having diabetes has made me realize I can't do everything, and it's ok to say no and not feel guilty. But I make myself take time for me and do what is good for me. I want to be around long enough to spoil my grandchildren.*

Stella Biggs says that one of her biggest challenges is keeping her low blood sugars from scaring her children. It's most difficult when her husband travels for work. She narrates:

> *[When lows happen] my husband says, "Mommy is silly right now." Most of the time it is when we are on vacation and away from reality that this happens, but they still get scared. They are old enough now that they even ask me how my blood sugar is doing, and if I act even a little weird, they ask*

me to check my blood sugar. I know they are scared, but they also love me and want me to be around. The hardest thing is when my husband travels for business. I have to be extremely aware and careful that I do not get any low blood sugars because I am the only one taking care of them at that time, and I don't want them to have to take care of me. I have been lucky so far that it has not gotten to the point of losing control, especially now, since I have my [continuous glucose monitoring] CGM, but before I had it, I was checking all hours of the night to make sure I was ok. Another challenging part of motherhood and diabetes is exercise. I work full time and then I have to juggle dinner, homework, and baths, plus spend quality time with my husband. I have been going to the gym at 5 AM to try and fit in exercise, but then I am so tired at night that I don't get to spend enough time with my husband. If I go to the gym after work, then I have to juggle the low blood sugars at the gym. It has been very challenging to find time with work and motherhood/marriage[and] to make time for exercise, which I clearly need.

Balancing work and motherhood is challenging for any mother. Making time for anything beyond work and home is very challenging, such as exercise, doctors' appointments for 3 people, birthday parties, etc. That is not exclusive to diabetic mothers, but we may have more doctors' appointments for ourselves than most mothers do; also, we can't skip the gym if we don't feel like it or the day gets too long at work.

Michelle Sorensen believes that her health needs to come first so she can be a healthy mother and someday, a healthy grandmother. She says, "However, at times, it is hard in the moment to put my needs first. For example, if I need to check my sugar but I have a crying newborn or whining toddler, it is hard to control my impulse to soothe my child first."

UNDERSTANDING GENETIC RISKS

When I was diagnosed in 1985, my doctor couldn't tell me why I'd gotten sick. My sister had been diagnosed 6 months earlier, and he said it was rare to have two diagnoses in the same family, especially so close together. I was told that diabetes ran in families. I remember that it felt like there was an element of blame between my parents, as if they were secretly wondering whose fault it was, and which one of them had the faulty genes. I remember that after I was diagnosed, people would ask how I got it and where it came from and feeling like there was something missing because I couldn't answer. Like a car crash, I wanted to be able to point at the source of my illness: the icy patch that made the car slip off the road, forever altering the course of my life. Other people wanted me to show them the crash too, so they could understand where it came from and reassure themselves that the same thing wouldn't happen to them. But I couldn't and 25 years later, I still can't.

STATISTICS

- A child born to a woman with type 1 diabetes who is younger than 25 years has a 1 in 25 risk of developing diabetes.
- If the child was born after the mother turned 25, his or her risk is 1 in 100.
- Your child's risk is doubled if you developed diabetes before the age of 11.
- If both you and your partner have type 1 diabetes, the risk is between 1 in 10 and 1 in 4.
- If a woman has type 2 diabetes, the risk of her child getting diabetes is 1 in 7 if she was diagnosed before the age of 50, and 1 in 13 if she was diagnosed after the age of 50.
- Other tests can also make your child's risk clearer. A special test that tells how the body responds to glucose can tell which school-aged children are most at risk.
- Another more expensive test can be done for children who have siblings that have type 1 diabetes. This test measures antibodies to insulin, to islet cells in the pancreas, or to an enzyme called glutamic acid decarboxylase. High levels can indicate that a child has a higher risk of developing type 1 diabetes.

Miles was drinking the bathwater again. I saw him as I walked by the open door of the bathroom, on my way to get the boys' pajamas from their bedroom. My feet dragged. The end of our long day would be over once I completed baths, jammies, books, and bed; then I could collapse onto the couch and read. I was almost there. But Miles was scooping water with a plastic bath toy, leaning his head forward, and sipping from the rim of the boat. The edges of his hair were wet and sticking to his cheeks.

"What are you doing?" I asked my then 4-year-old child, reaching to brush the wet hair from his face.

"I don't know," he said.

"Are you thirsty? Don't drink the bathwater, it's yucky. I'll get you something to drink." I walked into the kitchen, suddenly alert. With a sippy cup of chocolate milk in my hands, I wrapped Miles in a towel, handed him his chocolate milk, and watched as he gulped it down.

"Done," he said, handing it back to me empty.

Miles loves chocolate milk, apple juice, juice boxes, lemonade, and even water. He drinks quickly and often, and it scares me.

I remember being thirsty. I remember standing under the too-bright-middle-of-the-night lights of my private school dorm bathroom and gulping water from someone else's plastic cup. I was so thirsty that I'd been dreaming about water. So I pushed back my warm comforter and stood, weak and dizzy in the lonely darkness, finally, temporarily asleep, and drank another cup of water. Two days later, I was diagnosed with type 1 diabetes.

I remember a conversation that I had with my ob-gyn when I was pregnant with my first son, Will. I'd asked her about the chances of passing diabetes on to my children. She told me that they were slim, 1 in 100. "The chances were worse for fathers," she said, "1 in 17." I was glad that I was not a man. She explained that medical advances had turned a formerly fatal illness into a chronic disease, and the advances in research had prevented long-term complications.

From my mother, I inherited the color of my skin, my hair, and the shape of my mouth; whereas my long legs and the slope of my nose, I inherited from my dad. My children at 7 and 4 years old are now losing their teeth and learning to read. My blood is running through their bodies. Will has my nose and shoulders, and Miles looks like a younger me when his hair is long and with curls around his cheeks. Will is patient, and they both have a natural athleticism like their dad and this makes me confident that they will be accepted in their school's athletic teams because of the way they can run, jump, and throw. But I worry that they will have my introverted tendencies and I can already see my bad sense of direction in Will every time he walks out the front door. I hope that they are readers and lovers of books, but what about their genes? What will they inherit from me?

The next morning, as Miles sat at the kitchen's counter, watching cartoons and waiting for breakfast, I reached for his hand and explained that I was going to prick his finger. He didn't refuse, so I grabbed the tip of his index finger. Acting quickly so he wouldn't have time to pull away, I pinched the small, soft tip of his finger between my larger, calloused fingers. I pressed the Accu-Check against his skin, looking up once to reassure him, and then pushed the plunger. Pressing below the spot where I'd pricked, I collected a small, bright red dot of blood onto a test strip. Holding the machine in my hands, I waited.

After 5 seconds, the result showed up, Miles' blood sugar was 81. Worry evaporated from my body, and letting it go, I realized I'd been clenching my teeth. We were safe, for now.

When Your Kids Have Diabetes

When Sarah Howard's son was diagnosed with type 1 diabetes, he was only 23 months old. Sarah recalls:

> *When my youngest was diagnosed, it was the first time I was really thankful to have type 1 myself. I knew what to expect, but just had to learn how to manage it in a toddler. If it had all been new, it would have been much more overwhelming. It was still devastating, but not as overwhelming. We just make management part of normal life.*
>
> *I had noticed he'd been thirsty for about a week. But he was acting normally, not tired, so I didn't really think he had diabetes. (When I got it, I was so tired . . .). Then one night, he nursed all night long, it seemed, and then as soon as he got up he grabbed the water bottle and started carrying it around the house. I thought, ok, I should test him. But I didn't want to prick his little finger. My husband said, "just test him and you'll stop worrying about it." So that evening, after dinner, we tested him. The meter just said, "HI"—it didn't even give a number. I said, we've got to go to the ER. So we did—their finger prick came back as*

"critically high." They had to get a blood draw in order to even figure out his blood sugar—it was 798. But he didn't have ketoacidosis—probably due to such a sudden onset. (It's more sudden in younger children; I'd had symptoms for months before diagnosis). Afterwards, I realized he had been peeing a lot, at night, and he'd been dry at night in the past. Also, he'd been eating a lot, which I had attributed to a growth spurt. So, the symptoms were there, but I only noticed the thirst. I was looking for other symptoms that he didn't have. In any case, we stayed in the hospital that night, and were able to leave the next afternoon.

Since I already understood diabetes, the education was easier. I got the paperwork started for a pump that day. I do remember being thankful that he had diabetes, and not cancer. I knew I could manage it, that he'd survive, and have a semi-normal life at least. It could have been worse. Two days later, we finally got his blood sugar below 200 for the first time and I panicked again; how would I know if he was low? He couldn't talk! How would I survive this stress? It's gotten easier as he's gotten older.

I think it really helps that I have type 1, in how my child deals with it. I don't treat him differently, I don't think of him differently, etc. It's normal, he doesn't feel different, dealing with diabetes is just something we both have to do. He has to get poked, and so do I. I also totally understand what he is feeling and going through and that makes parenting easier for me. However, I was adult-onset, so I didn't have to go through childhood, puberty, or early adulthood with the disease. So I won't understand issues specific to those times of life. We definitely eat healthier food and exercise, but I did before diabetes, so I don't think it made much difference in lifestyle.

BENEFITS OF BEING A DIABETIC MOM

Rachel Garlinghouse believes that diabetes has made her a better person and a better mother. She says, "Diabetes gave me the motivation to learn about going green, making better food choices, exercising more, writing about my experiences, reaching out to others, and making new friends. I'm not going to pretend life with diabetes is all hearts and roses, because it's not, but for the most part, it has blessed me in ways I never would have imagined."

Cheryl Alkon says that she is trying hard to feed her son as healthily as possible, so he will establish lifelong healthy eating habits. She says:

> *He's not big on candy, mostly because I don't have it in the house and don't give it to him (he didn't eat any of his Halloween candy, even though he loved trick or treating). He also doesn't like the taste of juice, and therefore, doesn't want my juice boxes when I'm treating a low. I think my way of eating day-to-day has had an effect on him; he only drinks milk and water, as I do, and scrapes the icing off a piece of birthday cake because he thinks it's too sweet. He also likes oatmeal, which I ate everyday for breakfast while I was pregnant with him.*

Michelle Sorensen says:

> *Over the last 12 years with diabetes, my approach to health and well-being has really evolved. I now see stress management and relaxation as much more important. I consult with a naturopath and incorporate lots of different elements into my health management: nutrition, exercise, and positive thinking. So I absolutely believe that my knowledge and awareness means I have protected my children's health. If they are sick, I never send them back to daycare or school until they are completely back to normal because I am so protective of their immune systems. I use supplements to strengthen their systems and feed them the healthiest food I can.*

SINGLE PARENTING

Andrea McDowell is a single mom to her daughter Frances. She says that single parenthood has not been as difficult as she feared:

> *Every day I do the dishes by hand in the kitchen sink because the new apartment that I moved to with my daughter this summer does not have a dishwasher.*

My daughter sleeps upstairs in her new pink room with the red flowers I painted on the wall, her arms wrapped around a sleep-time friend, while downstairs, I put into practice those lessons from Home Ec so long ago—glass, then silverware, then dishes, then pots. I suspect I am the only one from that class to be doing so, if only because I am likely to be the only one who does not have a dishwasher.

The dishes done, the floor swept, the worst of the mud mopped from the front entryway, the toys returned to their rightful places, the school paperwork read over and dealt with appropriately, the kitchen table wiped, the counters scrubbed, and the leftovers refrigerated, I finally have 5 free minutes. Immediately, a thought intrudes; my insulin pump told me to change my infusion site 3 hours ago. Oops. I'd better do that now before I forget again.

I never forgot, before, when I was married. I never forgot to test or bolus or change my infusion site. I never went high for days on end because the time was always there to check my sugars after meals.

The infusion site is changed. Now, I have 5 free minutes. Real ones. Frances cries. I go upstairs to soothe her. So much for that.

Many things about single motherhood turned out to be surprising, mostly in good ways. For instance, it's not anywhere near as hard as I had feared. Frances is a preternaturally easy-going child who demands a lot of affection and attention but rewards this by never having thrown a temper tantrum. I had thought the separation might cause her to regress—that she would need diapers again, maybe, or become angry or sad or sullen, but no. There is a lot of work to do and it frequently takes every-thing I have in me to get it all done every day, but my little girl, thank the gods, seems to be handling it well.

Losing the house was also not traumatic. We have considerably less than half the space we used to and, commensurately, considerably less than half the stuff.

It's fine. I don't miss it. I never liked lawn maintenance and I'm just as happy not to have to shovel a driveway or clean snow from the car in the winter. Empty space is just an invitation to spend money to fill it, so far as I'm concerned. Here, in our new little nest, I sit on the couch with the computer and watch Frances play with her toys beside me on the floor. It's cozy, I think. I don't have cable, since I can't afford it, which gives us more time to spend together.

It's lovely to live one subway stop from my office, to know that Frances is that close when she is at school, to spend so little time commuting, to be able to walk or ride my bike when the weather is nice and get in some extra exercise. It's lovely to ride on the subway and be able to forget for weeks at a time that I even own a car. It's especially lovely, although expensive, to have a nice big bookstore right across the street. These are reasons that I chose to move us here, of course, but I hadn't expected to like them quite so much.

But then, there are surprises that can't be described as lovely, such as there is no slack when you are a single mother. Married moms can [act carelessly] in ways that you can't. You are already assumed to be screwing your kids up just because you do not have a husband; you are under more scrutiny and more suspicion, or at least, it feels like it. Things you would never have done when you were married, you do now, even though you have so much less time and energy, because you are single and you need to prove to the world that you can do this. You are not damaging the most important person in your world. He or she will be fine and you will be fine and you can handle all of this. I never mopped when I was married. I changed the sheets on a seasonal schedule when I was part of a couple; and now, it is regular as clockwork, every 2 weeks. Sometimes, when I was married, Frances would watch more than the 2 hours of television—that was our theoretical limit for a day. Now? Never. Sometimes, when I was married, her dinner was pasta from a can. Now? Every dinner she has eaten in my new home has been made by me, from scratch, except for carrot soup.

I wonder if this is why single motherhood is so much more exhausting than the partnered kind. We have no permission to slack off, ever. Not from the world, and not from ourselves.

She continues:

I was not surprised to read in the only medical study I found on the subject that single mothers with diabetes have significantly worse blood sugar control than married ones. Hey, I test when I can, I eat well, I exercise almost every day, and sometimes, that's already more than I can handle.

Just now, I looked down and realized that while I'd remembered to put the new infusion site in, I'd forgotten to take the old one out, so I was sporting one on each side of my stomach. A matched set. I can keep up with the big things but the details get away from me sometimes.

There is an incongruity here—I cannot afford cable, I do not have a dishwasher, but I have an insulin pump. Yes. I have health insurance that, lucky me, covers the cost of the pump and the supplies and insulin and test strips to 80%; even so, what's left over costs more than cable would. I sometimes think of that money and what I would do with it if I didn't need to spend it on keeping myself alive. Maybe, I'd save more for my retirement. Maybe, Frances and I would travel sometimes. Maybe, I'd spend it all on books. I very likely would still not have cable. It would be a lot more fun, whatever it is, than filling out paperwork to get myself reimbursed, and sticking myself with pins.

But the money is not what gets me. I've been paying for diabetes and its associated paraphernalia since I was 17 years old, and I just assume it now; it's in the budget, along with rent and groceries. Diabetes is, I've often observed, an expensive habit. It would be nice if Canada's stated commitment to socialized health care extended to those of us with chronic illnesses, but I don't expect it to, and neither do most of my acquaintances. I pay for it, and thank the powers that be that I have health insurance to reimburse me afterwards.

It isn't even the time. Testing, refilling cartridges, changing sites—none of these are time-consuming in and of themselves. It's when the time is. It's the competition for that time with a certain small girl who needs me, because when she is here, I am the only one she has. It's the keeping track. That insulin pump vibrates all day and night to remind me of what I need to do, and still, it's not enough. I still forget. I take the vibrating pump out of my pocket, check it, make a note to follow up as soon as this next task is over with—but then that task turns into another and another and hours have passed and I've forgotten. Frances's needs won't wait, and I tell myself that diabetes will, at least for a few minutes until I get her settled again—and then.

You will tell me, of course, that I can't take care of my daughter unless I take care of my diabetes, and in the abstract, that too is absolutely correct. In reality, in the particular moment when each choice is made (to test or delay, serve juice or change a site, find a toy or eat the snack I bolused for), my daughter's needs are more vocal and insistent. My mute pancreas cannot compete. Its technological handmaiden lacks large blue eyes and emphatic hugs. It doesn't love me, obviously, even though it takes care of me.

This does not prevent the potential consequences from presenting themselves to me late at night—what if I fall into a diabetic coma while I sleep and, one morning, my daughter wakes to find me in my bed, unable to wake? What would she do? She is too young to feed herself or get a drink, or open the door, and go for help. She can't use the toilet on her own. What would she do? How can I prepare her? There isn't a friend or family member I would choose to burden with the task of being my diabetes monitor, making sure I am conscious and coma-free. Whatever we do has to be something we can do, just the two of us.

So I force myself into a standard of motherhood I never even would have attempted before. The house clean, the meals all healthy and balanced, the toys wholesome, the television limited, everything perfect and in place on the outside. Yet underneath, what you won't see are the forgotten tests, the missed boluses, the infusion sets left in for an extra day or two, the guessed carb counts for meals. Everything looks perfect, though—happy daughter, competent mother, acceptable house; all powered by a neglected medical condition.

My arms are full, and that's the problem; too many things I carry (the job, the daughter, the house) cannot be dropped, even for a moment, because I am running as hard as I can to stay in place. The job, the daughter, the house—even for healthy women, single motherhood can be overwhelming, I know, so why should it be any different for me? My arms are full, and I'm running as fast as I can. Sometimes, something drops and it's almost always the diabetes—a test, a site, a bolus. They add up, I know and it's not my intention, but if I stop to pick it up, I'll only fall behind. I keep running, and tell myself I'll go back for them later.

AUTHENTIC ADVICE

- Rachel Garlinghouse says:
  Ladies, it is ok to say no. Be selective in what you do in life. Decide what matters most to you and pursue it with all your heart and energy. My priorities are my health, my family, my spiritual life, and my writing. I have secondary priorities like spending time with girlfriends and teaching. Anything else that tries to steal my focus and my joy is rejected without apology. Be strong, be confident, and most of all, say no often!
- Cheryl Alkon says:
  That airplane advice of taking care of yourself before being able to help others is a good one. As I heard recently, if your kids are young and want your attention, you don't need to drop everything if you need to do something crucial for yourself first. They're "crying, not dying," so if you need to take a moment to test your

blood sugar or suck down a juice box or glucose tabs amid the (nonemergency) crying, go ahead and don't feel guilty about it.

■ Cara Bauer says:

Enjoy every moment, it goes by so quickly. Take care of yourself as much as you take care of your baby. You want to be a happy, healthy mom for the baby you worked so hard to bring into this world.

■ Stella Biggs says:

Motherhood is difficult for any new mother, but having diabetes is not the end of the world. Just make sure you always keep snacks, juice, etc. in your diaper bag so that you can take care of yourself if need be. Use the alarms on the sensor to check your blood sugar, check if you are low/high. It is so easy to forget to eat or take insulin when you have a newborn. Just make it a part of your routine, because if you don't, you won't be around to watch that beautiful baby grow up. It may be difficult, but there are so many amazing women out there who have done this and succeeded, including me!

■ Michelle Sorensen says:

I would suggest viewing the diabetes as another child . . . a major responsibility that you have to learn to balance with newfound parental responsibilities. I firmly believe that if you put your health first, everything else will fall into place. If you lose your health, then you risk losing enjoyment of all those other things you put before your diabetes: career, family, etc. . . . However, attending to diabetes does not mean worrying about it all the time or berating yourself for the inevitable ups and downs. I try to have a short memory for my perceived failures—I learn from mistakes, correct [them], and move on. I let myself feel good about the good days, the good readings, the health changes I make . . . because positive emotions lead to more motivation and energy.

■ Sarah Howard says:

Give your children vitamin D, omega 3 fatty acids, and probiotics. All of these may help prevent type 1 in children. I've devoted myself to trying to figure out the environmental causes of type 1, and made a website to help other mothers in my position (who want to prevent their kids from getting type 1), www.diabetesandenvironment.org

Motherhood is one of the many adventures along the path of life. My first child was born on August 28, 2001. I tell him the story of his birth on the eve of his birthday every year, just like my mother tells me mine. I tell him how my feet were so swollen that they hurt to touch, how the sun was white and flat in the sky, and that the heat felt like Saran Wrap around my legs. I tell him how his dad and I drove to the hospital and checked ourselves in. How I spent the first night there alone and how, the next morning, I was hooked up to IVs and monitors and labored for over 2 hours. I edit the part about how the drugs, the pushing, the vacuum, and forceps couldn't get him out, how he had to be cut from my body. I tell him the part about hearing his cry, how something split apart inside of me with that sound, the sound of my child. He was here, I was a mother, and that was all that mattered.

That was almost 10 years ago and so much has changed. I am now a mother to three healthy boys. Since I became a mother, my husband hasn't reached over in the middle of the night to feel my sweaty back, to wake from the heaviness of sleep and rush to the kitchen for a glass of juice. Since I became a mother, he hasn't had to hold my head up and pour the juice into my mouth to try and bring me back. Becoming a mother has taught me how to take care of myself. It has also taught me that I am not alone.

There are other mothers, like myself, who kick their legs as they try to keep the weight of diabetes from pulling them to the murky bottom. Together, we are mothers with illnesses who bake dinners for teacher appreciation week, drive to t-ball practice, tennis lessons, arrange play-dates, drop our kids off at school, commute to work, and rock our babies until they fall back to sleep. We are mothers who test blood sugar levels, give shots, take medications, and arrange for doctor visits. Most of all, we are mothers who are caught in the familiar balancing act of work, raising a family, and finding time for ourselves and for our partners. What makes us different is the highs and lows of living with diabetes.

11 Aging Gracefully

The life expectancy of women living with diabetes used to be precariously low. Today, advances in health care have increased life spans, but as women with diabetes age, our risks for complications, such as heart disease, increase. However, it's not all doom and gloom. Whenever I start to think about my future and feel panicky, I think of the sage advice from Dr. Colwell, my endocrinologist who told me that as long as I was keeping my blood sugars as close to "normal" as possible, I didn't have to worry about complications.

The Centers for Disease Control and Prevention (CDC) report, *Diabetes and Women's Health Across the Life Stages*, states that as women age out of their reproductive years into their middle years, they experience major shifts in their social roles. For many women, these changes include the transition from childbearing to child-rearing, returning to full participation in the labor force, and often coping with sole responsibility for their households. These are also the years in which women's health issues include the effects of prolonged exposure to biological and behavioral risk factors acquired in adolescence and young adulthood. Specifically, factors such as prepregnancy weight, gestational weight gain and water retention, gestational diabetes, and low levels of physical activity that continue from young adulthood increase the women's risk of developing diabetes in midlife. This is also the period of life when some women experience the diminution in their physical and psychological health that may be associated with the menopause. Circumstances, such as past discontinuity in employment, separation, divorce, and widowhood, may make middle-aged women vulnerable to low family incomes and inadequate health care coverage, so that they may forego needed services, including preventive care for serious diseases such as diabetes.

STATISTICS

- The prevalence of diabetes doubles as women age out of the reproductive years into the middle years.
- For middle-aged women, diabetes is at least twice as common among nonwhites as among whites.
- Diabetes is the leading cause of death among middle-aged American women.
- A1c awareness: 64.5 percent of persons aged 30–44 years reported undergoing hemoglobin A1c (HbA1c) monitoring, compared with only 37.1 percent of persons aged 45–64 years and 10.6 percent of persons aged 65 years or older.

DIFFERENT PERSPECTIVES ON LIVING WITH AN ILLNESS

Jessica Bernstein has lived with type 1 diabetes since she was a child. Her documentary film, *Blood and Honey*, illustrates the ways various cultures view illness. Her film asks the question, "How can everyone benefit from the wisdom of those who have spent years learning how to live well in the face of suffering?" Jessica says that she has always had erratic blood sugars and that as a child she never rebelled, always participated in her care, and spent her childhood and teen years feeling guilty. One of her doctors used to send Jessica "report cards" with the results of her A1c, and she would check off: good, bad, and needs improvement. Jessica says, "It was torturous for me. These cards were so upsetting to me that I used to burn them when they arrived, that was the level of upset. It was upsetting for me to be in this category of the bad patient."

It wasn't until Jessica was in her 20s that she began to reflect on this part of her life and started to look at the judgment within the medical community. Jessica's PhD dissertation looked at identity development in people who had lived with diabetes since they were 5 years old, and found that almost every person had similar negative experiences with health care professionals. Respondents avoided doctors and created issues with authority figures. Their experiences created a deep distrust and the health care professionals wouldn't believe them and would sometimes reprimand them for lying. Patients were saying, "I'm doing everything you're telling me to do and it's not working. I don't need answers from doctors, I want empathy. When you have blood sugars that are out of wack, it's always assumed to be within your control. There is an imbalance of power with doctors and patients."

Jessica attempted for years to work within the system. She wrote letters to her doctors, but says the medical establishment realized they had nothing to offer her; they had no answers for her erratic blood sugars. Today, she works with non-Western practitioners and says that she has been treated with more respect and dignity: "When I go to see my Chinese doctor, he's looking at the bigger picture of my health and asking, 'How's your sleep?' 'How's your energy level?' because he is addressing the whole body."

In the research for her film, Jessica had worked with groups of disabled people and said that she has learned a different perspective on living with chronic illness.

Just because I'm not living a normal life doesn't mean I'm not living a rich and more meaningful life. People with diabetes don't want to think that they are different, so they put themselves in a different category than other chronic disabilities, which denies us access to people who have valuable knowledge and insight to how to live with disease. The reality is that these are [the] people that are living every day having to confront these issues that everybody has to deal with whether it's emotional or physical. We need to turn to these people and ask them what they've learned about life through suffering.

Jessica talks about these ideas in her film and website of the same name, *Blood and Honey,* and explains that a diagnosis in the African tribe is not seen as a tragedy, but as an initiation to a new phase of growth. "In order to make it through the crisis toward growth, you have to draw on community elders and ritual and that's what we're lacking in America."

It's a new way to look at living with chronic illness. "We talk about battling diabetes, but then you're battling yourself."

Judith Jones Ambrosini was diagnosed in 1962 at the age of 18 years and spent many years "fumbling through diabetes in unenlightened decades." Today, she is an active participant in "the present high-tech cyberspace era" and says that all the fluctuations in between have caused complications. She says:

> *Although I am in excellent general health (with a little arthritis), I have had a few bumps and bruises along the sugar road. In 1975, I went through a rather scary time with proliferative retinopathy. Lasers were still very new and technology was minimal. Luckily, I found a healer in Dr. Charles Campbell at the Harkness Eye Institute at Columbia Presbyterian Hospital in New York City. He saved my eyes. I have met many physicians over the years, but only a few I consider healers. Dr. Campbell was the first. As a result of all the powerful laser and cryotherapies when I was diagnosed, along with good diabetes management, my eyesight still serves me well today. There are a few reminders left such as poor night vision, poor left peripheral vision, and shaky depth perception. These things, though, are a small price to pay and a petty inconvenience.*
>
> *Having these complications snapped me into attention about managing diabetes. Because of improved management, I get good reports every year when I go for my retina checkup. When you develop a complication, it's like biting into a reality sandwich. These complications exist, but by doing our best to approach diabetes in a positive way and follow the guidelines of balance, there is a sense of success.*
>
> *I still think I'm 35! Every so often I realize I'm not. Getting older means waking up in the morning with the same sense of adventure and possibilities for the day that I always had. The only difference is I go to bed earlier at night. I look around at friends and others my age, and am very proud that diabetes has taught me to stay fit, eat a healthy diet, live in moderation, and love life.*

Linda Frick was diagnosed when she was 8 years old and has lived with diabetes for 50 years. She says:

> *I've had what I would consider some minor complications that started after the birth of my first child. It affects my tendons in my hands. They have thickened to the point of*

causing pain and complications with my everyday living. Just as I enter my 50th year of living with diabetes, I have had a major complication with my eyes. I've been told for years that I have had cataracts behind the lens of both eyes. They have never bothered me or impaired my ability to see clearly until most recently. I've seen a specialist who tells me they can successfully remove these cataracts. I know now that they do these operations on thousands of people with and without diabetes. Thankfully, I do not have any retinopathy in my eyes. I can remember years ago this same complication would cause blindness. I'm so thankful that the advancement of medical science has come at least this far. Of course, I would prefer a cure for my disease; however, I've seen great changes in how to keep my life as normal as possible. My complications have not changed my life. I have worked outside of my home in order to procure insurance benefits for myself and my family and joke to my colleagues that I will most likely die there at work on my computer.

Linda says that the greatest challenge that faces women with diabetes as they age is getting insurance to pay for the things that they need to survive. She adds:

The insurance companies keep reducing their coverage. Drug companies also make huge profits from supplies that we need to survive, such as test strips and pump supplies. The costs keep escalating. I also think that depression can be something to be very aware of for us diabetics. The news of complications can be devastating. For those without insurance coverage, it can be the difference between good control and poor control. I can attest that we've come a long way in the last 50 years, but I worry about our nation's current economic situation and how it will affect our ability to stay healthy in these times.

Linda has seen a lot of changes in her 50 years with diabetes. She recalls, "When I was first diagnosed, the medical community didn't think anyone with diabetes could live past their 30th birthday. With lots of hard work, I've beaten those odds and rejoice that I'm still here to prove them wrong! I've been rewarded by having a family (I was advised not to), by keeping a full time job (I was denied my first job due to my disease back in the early 1970s—this was before equal opportunity rights), and by doing what I love best—traveling."

DIET AND EXERCISE

The CDC report states that the interventions to increase physical activity in this population may significantly improve glycemic control, particularly in older, physically inactive women, who are at increased risk for developing diabetes. It says, "Increased physical activity can also reduce the risk of coronary heart disease (CHD), the leading cause of death among women with diabetes. A 35-55 percent reduction in risk for CHD is associated with maintaining an active lifestyle."

Linda Frick says that losing weight has been a huge benefit for both feeling better and staying healthy. "In my late 30s and 40s, I had gained 20 pounds that caused me to feel horrible. I have since lost that weight and can really feel the difference just like between night and day!"

MENOPAUSE

In "Menopause: What to Expect, How to Cope," Pat Dougherty, CNM, MSN, and Joyce Green Pastors, MS, RD, CDE, wrote that menopause can be especially challenging for women with diabetes.[1]

> *For most women, menopause—the cessation of menstrual periods—is a normal or natural occurrence. The average age at menopause is 51 years old, although any time after 40 years old is considered normal.*
>
> *Both the perimenopausal and postmenopausal periods may present additional challenges for women who have diabetes. For one thing, the hormonal fluctuations that are common to perimenopause can affect blood glucose levels. For another, some symptoms of menopause are the same as or easily confused with the symptoms of high or low blood glucose levels, so the cause must be determined before corrective action can be taken. In addition, both diabetes and menopause raise a woman's risk of osteoporosis, so women with*

diabetes must be proactive about taking steps to keep their bones strong. Lack of sleep, whether related to menopause, stress, or something else, can disrupt diabetes control. In addition, menopause is often associated with weight gain, which can make blood glucose control more difficult.

The unstable levels of estrogen and progesterone contribute to menstrual cycle irregularities and perimenopausal symptoms. They can also contribute to unstable blood glucose levels. Although the effects of estrogen and progesterone on diabetes control are not entirely understood in general, it appears that higher levels of estrogen may improve insulin sensitivity, whereas higher levels of progesterone may decrease insulin sensitivity. When insulin sensitivity decreases, more insulin is needed to get glucose into the cells.

One of the challenges for menopausal women who have diabetes is distinguishing between the symptoms of the two conditions. It is not uncommon to mistake menopause-related hot flashes or moodiness for symptoms of low blood glucose. Night sweats—hot flashes that occur at night—can interrupt sleep and lead to excessive daytime fatigue, which can also be mistaken for low blood glucose. If this leads to eating extra calories to raise a low blood glucose level, it could lead to high blood glucose and, over time, weight gain, if repeated on a regular basis.

Regular blood glucose monitoring can help women figure out whether low or high blood glucose levels may be causing their symptoms.

Lifestyle changes are always the first step to help reduce the discomforts of menopause. The following changes can help make the menopausal transition easier:

- *Remain (or become) physically active. Regular physical activity or exercise can help increase energy levels, improve mood, and combat weight gain.*

- *Substitute whole grains and fresh fruits and vegetables for processed and refined foods, both to help control blood glucose (and blood pressure) levels and to increase overall energy level.*

- *Use alcohol and caffeine in moderation or not at all, because they can trigger hot flashes and decrease sleep quality. If spicy foods have a similar effect, reduce your intake or avoid them altogether.*

- *Consume more legumes (beans and peas), soy foods, and flaxseed. These foods contain* phytoestrogens—*chemicals found in plants that may act like estrogen in the body. Some women report that increasing the amounts of these foods in their diet decreases the frequency and severity of their hot flashes, although scientific studies have not confirmed this. (Phytoestrogen pills and powders are not recommended at this time because of safety concerns.)*

- *Get adequate amounts of vitamins and minerals. To keep their bones strong, women going through menopause who are not receiving hormone therapy should be getting 1,200–1,500 milligrams of calcium and 800 international units of vitamin D each day (which can be provided by three to four 8-ounce servings per day of low-fat milk or yogurt). Women receiving hormone therapy should aim for 1,000 milligrams of calcium per day. Vitamin E and the B vitamins have also been suggested as beneficial for reducing menopausal symptoms, but the research does not currently provide strong support.*

- *Use of herbal teas or supplements may be helpful for treating hot flashes and night sweats. Research is limited, but herbal preparations such as black cohosh, garden sage, and motherwort are used in many Asian and European countries. However, you should speak with your doctor before beginning any sort of herbal regimen.*

- *If you are a smoker, stop smoking.*

Because women with diabetes already have an increased risk of heart disease, it is especially important for women with diabetes to discuss the benefits and risks of herbal treatment with their health care providers. Heart disease is the leading cause of death among American women.

Perhaps the most important thing a perimenopausal woman can do is to listen to and respect her body. Just as each person's diabetes requires an individualized plan for control, so is each woman's experience with menopause unique. Because it's common to experience some changes in blood glucose control as you go through menopause, it helps to maintain a regular schedule of blood glucose monitoring, as well as good exercise and eating habits. Using relaxation techniques to reduce stress and trying to get adequate sleep can help too. Consult your health care provider if your symptoms are severe and are dramatically affecting your quality of life.

Brenda is 51 years old, has type 1 diabetes, and is dealing with menopause. She says that she has days where it's difficult to remember that menopause is a natural process that affects everyone differently, whether you have diabetes or not. She says:

After extensive research and discussions with my ob-gyn, MD, and certified diabetes educator (CDE) (all females in their 50s), I decided to treat my symptoms with bioidentical hormones (Vivelle-Dot estrogen patch and Prometrium tablets). I noticed a difference almost immediately—and have taken them regularly for a year. As much as I initially resisted the idea, at their suggestion, a few months ago, I also decided to try a low dose antidepressant. For those who don't feel comfortable with taking anything, believe me, I understand. I'm a massage therapist, and my first choice has always been a natural approach, and to avoid chemical intervention whenever possible. But the question became, why be miserable when you have other choices?

AUTHENTIC ADVICE

■ Judith Jones Ambrosini says:
  Smile. Laugh. Have lots of friends. Continue to learn about diabetes. Be involved with the things in life that make you happy. Don't worry.

■ Jessica Bernstein says:

The diabetes community has to come together, letter writing campaigns, and grassroots efforts to take "control" out of diabetes, the diabetes community has to come together . . . there is a power dynamic with doctors, it's a delicate thing.

■ Linda Frick says:

Take care of yourself first. Don't let any complications drag your morale down. Be thankful you have options for treatment nowadays. Keep up to date with medical knowledge so you can ask your doctor how it will affect your control. Be an optimist and it will help you win in the end. In my opinion, one of the most important things about aging with diabetes is to have an excellent working relationship with your doctor. I see an internal medicine doctor, and she refers me to an endocrinologist only when I need something that she can't help me with. We have a close doctor–patient relationship, and I trust her direction for my care. My advice is to shop around until you find the perfect fit for you.

Resources

BOOKS

Alkon, C. (2010). *Balancing pregnancy with pre-existing diabetes: Healthy mom, healthy baby.* New York, NY: Demos Health.

American Diabetes Association. (2001). *Diabetes & pregnancy: What to expect. Your guide to a healthy pregnancy and a happy, healthy baby.* Alexandria, VA: Author.

Bliss, A. (2007). *The discovery of insulin: Twenty-fifth anniversary edition.* Chicago, IL: University of Chicago Press.

Colberg-Ochs, S. (2001). *The diabetic athlete: Prescriptions for exercise and sports.* Champaign, IL: Human Kinetics.

Colberg-Ochs, S. (2006) *The 7 steps diabetes fitness plan: Living well and being fit with diabetes, no matter your weight.* New York, NY: Da Capo Press/Marlowe & Company.

Colberg-Ochs, S. (2009). *The diabetes athlete's handbook: Your guide to peak performance.* Champaign, IL: Human Kinetics.

Dominick, A. (1998). *Needles: A memoir of growing up with diabetes.* New York, NY: Touchstone.

Feudtner, C. (2003). *Bittersweet: Diabetes, insulin, and the transformation of illness.* Chapel Hill, NC: University of North Carolina Press.

Frank, A. W. (1995). *The wounded storyteller: Body, illness, and ethics.* Chicago, IL: University of Chicago Press.

Jovanovic-Peterson, L., Biermann, J., & Toohey, B. (1996). *The diabetic woman: All your questions answered.* New York, NY: Tarcher/Putnam.

Palmer, K. G. (2006). *When you're a parent with diabetes: A real-life guide to staying healthy while raising a family.* Hobart, NY: Hatherleigh Press.

Poirier, L. M., & Coburn, K. M. (2000). *Women and diabetes: Staying healthy in body, mind, and spirit* (2nd ed.). Alexandria, VA: American Diabetes Association.

Roszler, J., Polonsky, W. H., & Edelman, S. V. (2004). *The secrets of living and loving with diabetes: Three experts answer questions you've always wanted to ask.* Chicago, IL: Surrey Books.

Roszler, J., & Rice, D. (2007). *Sex and diabetes: For him and for her.* Alexandria, VA: American Diabetes Association.

Strotmeyer, E. S., Steenkiste, A. R., Foley, T. P., Jr., Berga, S. L., & Dorman, J. S. (2003). Menstrual cycle differences between women with type 1 diabetes and women without diabetes. *Diabetes Care, 26*(4), 1016–1021.

WEBSITES

American Association of Diabetes Educators: http://www.diabeteseducator.org

American Diabetes Association: http://www.diabetes.org

American Dietetic Association: http://www.eatright.org

Americans with Disabilities Act: http://www.ada.gov

Behavioral Diabetes Institute: http://www.behavioraldiabetesinstitute.org

Blood & Honey: http://www.bloodandhoney.org

Diabetes Forecast: http://www.fore.cast.org

Diabetes Health: http://www.diabeteshealth.com

Diabetes Mine: http://www.diabetesmine.com

Diabetes Sisters: http://www.diabetessisters.org

Exercise Is Medicine: http://exerciseismedicine.org

Insulinindependence: http://www.insulinindependence.org

Joslin Diabetes Center: http://www.joslin.org

The Center for Mindful Eating: http://www.tcme.org

Team WILD: Women Inspiring Life with Diabetes: http://www.teamwild.org

Test B4U Drive: http://www.medtronicdiabetes.com/testb4udrive/faqs

Transportation Security Administration (TSA) website provides extensive guidance on traveling with diabetes, including the following:

■ *Hidden Disabilities: Travelers with Disabilities and Medical Conditions:* http://www.tsa.gov/travelers/airtravel/specialneeds/editorial_1374.shtm

■ *Changes in Allowances for Persons with Disabilities at Airport Security Checkpoints:* http://www.tsa.gov/assets/pdf/special_needs_memo.pdf

■ *Travelers with Disabilities and Medical Conditions:* http://www.tsa.gov/travelers/airtravel/specialneeds/index.shtm

■ *Discrimination:* http://www.tsa.gov/travelers/customer/discrimination.shtm

The association also has more information on travel in general, not just security issues, such as the following:

■ *When You Travel:* http://www.diabetes.org/living-with-diabetes/treatment-and-care/medication/when-you-travel.html

TuDiabetes: *Traveling the world with diabetes.* Retrieved from http://www.tudiabetes.org/group/travelingtheworldwithdiabetes/forum

References

Facts and statistics from the Centers for Disease Control and Prevention report, *Diabetes and Women's Health Across the Life Stages*, are used throughout this book.

INTRODUCTION

1. Greenberg, R. (2010, May 27). Diabetes Health: Nicole Johnson, former Miss America, kicks off diabetes sisters' 1st "weekend for women." *Huffington Post*. Retrieved from http://www.huffingtonpost.com/riva-greenberg/diabetes-health-nicole-jo_b_589326.html.

CHAPTER 1: DIAGNOSIS

1. Frank, A. W. (1995). *The wounded storyteller: Body, illness, and ethics*. Chicago, IL: University of Chicago Press.
2. Kübler-Ross, E. (1969). *On death and dying*. New York, NY: Simon & Schuster.
3. Sparling, M. K. *Diabetes terms of endearment* (3rd ed.). Retrieved from http://sixuntilme.com/blog2/blogging_bits/.
4. Palmer, K. G. (2006). *When you're a parent with diabetes: A real life guide to staying healthy while raising a family*. Hobart, NY: Hatherleigh Press.

CHAPTER 2: MANAGING ADOLESCENCE

1. Maharaj, S., Daneman, D., Olmsted, M., & Rodin, G. (2004). Metabolic control in adolescent girls: Links to relationality and the female sense of self. *Diabetes Care, 27*(3), 709–715.
2. Wysocki, T. (2002). Parents, teens, and diabetes. *Diabetes Spectrum, 15*(1), 6–8. doi:10.2337/diaspect.15.1.6.
3. Joslin Diabetes Center. *Tips for safe driving*. Retrieved from http://www. joslin.org/phs/driving_with_diabetes.html.

CHAPTER 3: DIET

1. Bliss, M. (2007). *The discovery of insulin: Twenty-fifth anniversary edition* (pp. 150–151). Chicago, IL: University of Chicago Press.
2. Owens, M. D. (2003). Diabetes and women's health issues: Preface. *Diabetes Spectrum, 16*(3), 146–147. doi:10.2337/diaspect.16.3.146.
3. The Center for Mindful Eating. *The principles of mindful eating*. Retrieved from http://www.tcme.org/principle.htm.
4. American Diabetes Association. (n.d.). *Create your plate*. Retrieved from http://www.diabetes.org/food-and-fitness/food/planning-meals/create-your-plate/.
5. Bernstein, R. (2007). *Dr. Bernstein's diabetes solution: The complete guide to achieving normal blood sugars*. New York, NY: Little Brown and Company.

CHAPTER 4: EATING DISORDERS AND BODY IMAGE

1. Behavioral Diabetes Institute. Retrieved from http://www.behavioraldiabetes institute.org.
2. Park Nicollet. Retrieved from http://www.parknicollet.com/eatingdisorders/.
3. Center for Hope of the Sierras. Retrieved from http://www.centerforhope ofthesierras.com/.

CHAPTER 5: EXERCISE

1. National Eye Institute. *Facts About Diabetic Retinopathy*. Retrieved from http://www.nei.nih.gov/health/diabetic/retinopathy.asp.
2. Colberg-Ochs, S. (2008). *50 secrets of the longest living people with diabetes*. New York, NY: Marlowe & Company/Da Capo Books.
3. Colberg-Ochs, S. *Emotional fitness through physical activity*. Retrieved from http://www.shericolberg.com/exercise-columns9.asp.
4. Colberg-Ochs, S. (2001). *The diabetic athlete: Prescriptions for exercise and sports*. Champaign, IL: Human Kinetics.

CHAPTER 6: DATING, SEX, AND MARRIAGE

1. MicroMass Communications, Inc. (2010, December). A leader in behavioral marketing in the healthcare industry: New study reveals low sex drive in women with diabetes. *Medical News Today*. Retrieved from http://www.medicalnewstoday.com/articles/210676.php.
2. Trief, M. P. (2006, July 21). Diabetes and your marriage: Making things work. *Diabetes Self-Management*. Retrieved from http://www.diabetesselfmanagement.com/Articles/Emotional-Health/diabetes_and_your_marriage/1/.
3. Polonsky, W. (1999). *Diabetes burnout: What to do when you can't take it anymore*. Alexandria, VA: American Diabetes Association.

CHAPTER 7: WORKING GIRL: DIABETES AT WORK AND SCHOOL

1. Joffee, R. (2008). *Women, work, and autoimmune disease: Keep working, girlfriend*! New York, NY: Demos Health. Retrieved from http://diabetes.webmd.com/features/tips-to-help-you-manage-your-diabetes-at-work.

CHAPTER 9: PREGNANCY

1. Dunn, P. (2004). Perinatal lessons from the past, Dr Priscilla White (1900–1989) of Boston and pregnancy diabetes. *Archives of Disease in Childhood Fetal and Neonatal Edition, 89*, F276–F278. doi:10.1136/adc.2003.042739.

2. von Wartburg, L. (2007, July). Prevent birth defects: Don't get pregnant until your sugar is controlled. *Diabetes Health*. Retrieved from http://www. diabeteshealth.com/read/2007/07/14/5303/prevent-birth-defects-dont-get-pregnant-until-your-sugar-is-controlled.
3. Diabetes in Pregnancy Society. *Diabetes Australia*. Retrieved from http://www.adips.org.

CHAPTER 10: MOTHERHOOD

1. Buxton-Truffer, J. (2004) *Explaining chronic illness to your child*. Retrieved from http://bikecoc.nationalmssociety.org/site/DocServer/Winter_2004.pdf?docID =22041.
2. Howard, S. Teddy's story. *Diabetes forecast*. Retrieved from http://forecast. diabetes.org/magazine/reflections/teddys-story.
3. McDowell, A. (2009). Sugar mama. *Brain Child*. Retrieved from http://www. andreamcdowell.com/clips/brain_child_sugar_mama.pdf.

CHAPTER 11: AGING GRACEFULLY

1. Dougherty, P., & Green Pastors, J. (2008, March 4). Menopause: What to expect, how to cope. *Diabetes Self-Management*. Retrieved from http:// www.diabetesselfmanagement.com/Articles/Sexual-Health/menopause/.

Index